TRAUMA
NURSING
SECRETS

TRAUMA NURSING SECRETS

Sharon Saunderson Cohen, RN, MSN, CEN, CCRN

Trauma Clinical Nurse Specialist
Division of Trauma
North Broward Hospital District
Fort Lauderdale, Florida

HANLEY & BELFUS, INC.
An Affiliate of Elsevier

HANLEY & BELFUS, INC.
An Affiliate of Elsevier

The Curtis Center
Independence Square West
Philadelphia, Pennsylvania 19106

Disclaimer: This book is not intended to be prescriptive, but rather offers the collective wisdom of trauma nurses. Although the information in this book has been carefully reviewed for accuracy, neither the authors nor the editor nor the publisher can accept any legal responsibility for any errors. Neither the publisher nor the editor makes any warranty, expressed or implied, with respect to the material contained herein.

Library of Congress Control Number: 2002109094

TRAUMA NURSING SECRETS   ISBN 1-56053-518-0

Permissions may be sought directly from Elsevier's Health Sciences Rights Department in Philadelphia: USA: phone (+1) 215-238-7869, fax: (+1) 215-238-2239, e-mail: healthpermissions@elsevier.com. You may also complete your request on-line via the Elsevier homepage (http://www.elsevier.com), by selecting "Customer Support" and then "Obtaining Permissions."

Printed in the United States of America

Last digit is the print number: 9   8   7   6   5   4   3   2

CONTENTS

CONTRIBUTORS

Mary-Ellen Anton, RN, BSN, MHM, CCRN, CPTC
Organ Procurement Coordinator and Coordinator Supervisor, University of Miami Organ Procurement Organization, Miami, Florida

Sharon Saunderson Cohen, RN, MSN, CEN, CCRN
Trauma Clinical Nurse Specialist, Division of Trauma, North Broward Hospital District, Fort Lauderdale, Florida

Stephen M. Cohen, MS, PA-C, EdD (c)
Associate Professor and Assistant Dean, College of Allied Health, Nova Southeastern University, Fort Lauderdale, Florida

Jeanne Eckes-Roper, RN, BSPA-HCA
Clinical Director, Trauma Services, Broward General Medical Center, Fort Lauderdale, Florida

Cindy A. Garlesky, MSN, ARNP, CEN
Department of Preventive Medicine, Miami Children's Hospital, Miami, Florida

Steven D. Glow, RN, MSN, FNP, CEN, EMT-P
Nursing Faculty, Salish Kootenai College, Pablo, Montana; Emergency Department Nurse, Community Medical Center, Missoula, Montana; Critical Care Transport Nurse, Polson Emergency Services, Polson, Montana

Bobette G. Henslee, RN, BSN, CCRN
Outreach Coordinator, Trauma Services, Broward General Medical Center, Fort Lauderdale, Florida

Richard L. Herm, RN, BSN, CEN, CNRN
Research Nurse, Field Neurosciences Institute, Saint Mary's Hospital, Saginaw, Michigan

Cindy Jimmerson, RN
Research Investigator, National Science Foundation, Community Medical Center, Missoula, Montana

Patricia A. Manion, RN, MS, CCRN
Trauma Coordinator, Genesys Regional Medical Center, Grand Blanc, Michigan

Karen March, RN, MN, CNRN, CCRN
Clinical Faculty, Department of Biobehavioral Nursing and Health Systems, University of Washington, Seattle, Washington; Director of Clinical Development, Integra Neuroscience, San Diego, California

John J. Mason, RN, CEN, CFRN
Staff Nurse, Ryder Trauma Center, Miami, Florida

Donna M. Matthews, RN, BSN, CWOCN
Manager, Clinical Services, Pegasus Airwave, Inc., Boca Raton, Florida

Ruth Paiano, MS, ARNP
Adjunct Faculty, Health Sciences Division, Broward Community College, Fort Lauderdale, Florida; Director, Neurological Institute, North Broward Medical Center, Pompano Beach, Florida

Kristopher G. Pidgeon, RN, MSN, CEN
Clinical Nurse Specialist, Emergency Department, Memorial Regional Hospital, Hollywood, Florida

Joe Spillane, PharmD, ABAT
Associate Professor, Nova Southeastern University College of Pharmacy; Clinical Coordinator, Department of Pharmacy, Broward General Medical Center, Fort Lauderdale, Florida

FOREWORD

The organized chaos that follows the arrival of a trauma patient to the resuscitation room is perhaps the best example in medicine of the importance of a well-trained multidisciplinary team. Paramedics give their report while physicians, nurses, respiratory therapists, radiology technicians, phlebotomists, and others work diligently to save those precious minutes that may make the difference between life, death, or disability. Every member of the team has assigned tasks that are interdependent and based on a solid understanding of the pathophysiology affecting the trauma victim. Unfortunately, not many trauma textbooks have been written that target the nonphysician members of the team. In *Trauma Nursing Secrets*, the authors have been able to fill that need with an extremely useful and informational work.

The book is divided into four sections. Section I provides an overview of trauma systems, injury physiology, mechanics, and the prehospital approach. The chapters of Section II discuss forensics and injury prevention. Most important is a chapter focusing solely on medicine's newest challenge: weapons of mass destruction and bioterrorism. Throughout Section III, the authors present a system-by-system discussion of organ injuries and treatment. Finally, Section IV is a collection of some of the most challenging and intimidating problems facing trauma care providers, such as burns, pediatrics, and pregnancy.

As a colleague who has worked with many of the authors, I feel a sense of vicarious pride in their excellent accomplishment. As a consumer, I am most grateful for the readers committed to broadening their knowledge and expertise in caring for the injured. They will be pleased to find this book not only educational, but also entertaining.

Ivan Puente, MD, FACS
Clinical Assistant Professor of Surgery
Nova Southeastern University School of Medicine
Chief, Division of Trauma Services
Broward General Medical Center
Fort Lauderdale, Florida

PREFACE

The topics included in this book are based on answers to many of the questions that are asked of me by fellow nurses. I believe that no question is too simple, too complex, or unworthy of being asked. Most questions arise from a story, patient, or case, and many answers contain wonderful "secrets" of our profession. Trauma, like other disease states, is a specialty unto its own. My hope is that the pages of this book will answer some of the most common questions we all ask regarding the care we give to trauma patients. All the answers cannot be found in these pages, but then again neither can all the questions.

I could never have completed the task of editing this book without all the incredibly knowledgeable authors that contributed to it. Each of them is an expert and chose to share some of his or her knowledge, excitement for nursing, and professionalism with you, the reader. To each author, I give my special thanks for such an incredible job. In addition, Dr. Linda Scheetz, Nursing Secrets Series® editor, has guided the process of writing and editing from the beginning. I appreciate all her edits, reviews, comments, and direction. She is an editor's dream—especially mine.

As I complete the last details of this book, I realize how lucky I have been in my professional career to have in my life two women who have and continue to mentor and motivate me. From them, I have gained a passion for excellence, caring, and professionalism. Kim Kingsbury Osborne, RN, and Kathy King, ARNP, MSN, you are the best role models a novice or experienced nurse could ever want. I am blessed with your friendships, conversations, and examples.

To my husband, Steve, and daughter, Kierstin, words cannot tell you how much you mean to me. You have allowed me to spend many hours in front of the computer and away from you. Your love and support allowed this dream to be a reality.

Dad, although you are not here to see how big my smile is as I look at the finished product, it was you who gave me the writing bug and the silly idea that I could accomplish anything. I hope you can look down from heaven and smile with me. I love and miss you.

Sharon Saunderson Cohen, RN, MSN, CEN, CCRN

I. Clinical Management in Trauma Nursing

1. TRAUMA SYSTEMS: AN ORGANIZED APPROACH

Jeanne Eckes-Roper, RN, BSPA-HCA

1. Define trauma.

The word *trauma* is from the Greek root meaning "bodily injury." It is defined as a blunt or penetrating external force exerted on the body resulting in injury.

2. How long has trauma been a societal problem?

Traumatic injury is recognized as part of the human experience. Anthropologic studies of Neanderthal man have identified bodily injuries sustained during conflict. Although societal violence has not changed greatly since the early days of civilization, the incidence, cause, magnitude, and mechanisms of injury have changed significantly.

3. How has the military contributed to the development of trauma systems?

Military conflicts became the catalyst for the development of trauma care systems. Lessons learned on the battlefields have been incorporated into modern delivery of trauma care.

4. Why is there a need for organized trauma systems?

Trauma occurs in epidemic proportions in contemporary society. For each death due to trauma there are two known cases of disability. Unintentional injury is responsible for more deaths between the ages of 15 and 34 years than any other cause.

5. Define a trauma care system.

A trauma care system is defined as a health care delivery system that integrates and coordinates emergency medical services and hospital resources to provide optimal care that enhances positive patient outcomes.

6. Why provide a system rather than a trauma center?

No one trauma center can handle the problem alone. Allocations of resources within a system allow patients to receive the highest level of available care while avoiding excessive cost and inappropriate resource expenditure.

7. Why were trauma systems developed?

Trauma systems were developed to minimize the time from injury to definitive care management. In 1990 the Trauma Care Systems Planning and Development Act called for the development of a Model Trauma Care System Plan (MTCSP).

8. When were trauma systems first organized?

In 1992 the MTCSP became reality. The plan served as a framework for states to use as a template in designing trauma systems.

9. Describe inclusive and exclusive trauma systems.

Inclusive system	Exclusive system
All patients	Critically injured patients only
All providers	Level I and II trauma centers
All facilities	Typically in urban and suburban settings

Adapted from the Model Trauma Care System Plan. Rockville, MD, U.S. Department of Health and Human Services, 1992, with permission.

10. Describe an inclusive trauma system.

An inclusive system recognizes a variety of resources, including providers, institutions, and services, that provide care to patients in a comprehensive, integrated manner.

11. How are trauma systems considered inclusive?

The trauma center remains the critical link in a system that encompasses all phases of the continuum of care from resuscitation to rehabilitation. A trauma patient must be transported to a facility with appropriate resources that can provide high-quality care in a safe, efficient, and cost-effective manner.

12. Why is the inclusive system a better option?

All health care facilities, trauma centers, and acute care hospitals participate in providing optimal trauma care. Acute care hospitals are afforded the opportunity to consult and transfer to trauma centers in appropriate circumstances.

13. What are the key components in developing a trauma system?

- Leadership
- System development
- Legislation
- Finance

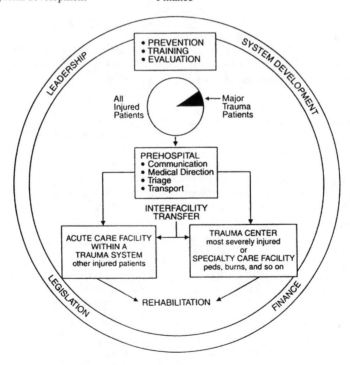

An inclusive trauma care system. (Adapted from the Model Trauma Care System Plan. Rockville, MD, U.S. Dept. of Health and Human Services; 1992, with permission.)

14. Categorize the challenges facing trauma system development.

Political
- State legislatures need to determine the need and establish a designating authority for trauma centers.
- Criteria for the system, triage, and transport protocols must be developed.
- Appropriate facilities must be identified to deliver care and oversight authority for performance improvement activities and system evaluation.

Economic
- Uncompensated care (patients are frequently underinsured or carry no insurance).
- Inadequate reimbursement by health maintenance organizations and third-party payors.
- Insufficient diagnosis-related group (DRG) payment schedules.

Professional
- Utilization and depletion of hospital resources by trauma patients.
- Trauma center designation is used as a status symbol in the community.
- Turf battles among disciplines and departments over diagnostic procedures and equipment.

Educational
- Basic, advanced, and continuing trauma education for all providers at all levels of care.
- Triage and transport protocols.
- Interfacility transfer agreements.

15. Explain the levels of trauma center care.

Resources for Optimal Care of the Injured Patient, published by the American College of Surgeons' Committee on Trauma (ACS-COT), identifies four levels of trauma center care:

Level I: regional resource trauma center/tertiary referral facility. This level of care is central to the trauma system and must provide the following:
- All aspects of care for injured patients
- Leadership in education, system development, research, and evaluation
- Commitment to education for all levels of providers, including first responders, emergency medical technicians, paramedics, nurses, and physicians
- Major community education outreach and injury prevention programs
- Comprehensive performance improvement plan to evaluate all aspects of care

Level II: community trauma center. Level II facilities are expected to provide the following:
- Initial definitive trauma care (patients with complex injuries may be transferred to a level I facility)
- Leadership role if no level I facility is located in the region
- Performance improvement plan to evaluate all aspects of care

Level III: rural trauma hospital. Level III facilities serve communities without ready access to level I or II trauma centers and must provide the following:
- Immediate emergency resuscitative care, emergent operations, and stabilization for transfer to a higher level of care or facility capable of providing definitive care
- Transfer agreements and protocols to expedite transfers
- Comprehensive performance improvement plan in place to evaluate all aspects of care

Level IV: facilities in remote areas. Level IV facilities must be able to provide the following:
- Advanced trauma life support
- Initial stabilization and preparation for transport to a higher level of care
- Transfer agreements and protocols to expedite transfers

16. How are patients selected for transport to trauma centers?

Patients are triaged to trauma centers by the emergency medical service (EMS) providers.

17. Define triage.

Triage is derived from the French word *triager* meaning "to sort."

18. What is the major goal of triage?

To match the injured patient with the most appropriate facility to limit morbidity and prevent mortality.

19. What systems have been developed for triage?

Prehospital personnel provide on-scene initial assessment and management. Triage guidelines are usually established on a local, regional, or state level.

20. Does triage occur only in the prehospital arena?

No. Triage continues as patients are reassessed in the trauma center.

21. What systems are used to triage trauma patients?

The two systems most commonly used to triage trauma patients are based on the acuity of the patient's condition and the need for medical attention: (1) emergent, urgent, and nonurgent and (2) levels I–V.

22. Define emergent, urgent, and nonurgent.

The **emergent** category includes patients with life- or limb-threatening injuries who require immediate interventions to prevent significant morbidity or mortality (e.g., gunshot wound to chest, motor vehicle collision resulting in significant hypotension, new-onset paralysis due to traumatic mechanism, fractures with vascular compromise).

The **urgent** category includes patients for whom definitive care may be delayed up to 2 hours without negative outcome (e.g., head trauma without loss of consciousness, extremity fractures without vascular compromise).

The **nonurgent** category includes injured patients who may wait for more than 2 hours for definitive care without a negative outcome (e.g., minor wounds, soft tissue injury, single bone fracture).

23. Explain levels I–V.

Level I: patients in critical condition who require immediate medical treatment (e.g., cardiac arrest, seizures, major multiple trauma, severe head injury).

Level II: unstable patients who need treatment initiated within 5–15 minutes (e.g., acute asthma attack, major fractures, attempted suicide, eye injury with loss of vision, pregnant women with active bleeding).

Level III: potentially unstable patients who require care within 30–60 minutes (e.g., drug intoxication, closed fracture, noncardiac chest pain, bleeding with stable vital signs).

Level IV: stable patients for whom care can be provided within 1–2 hours (e.g., minor burn, sore throat, strains and sprains, earache).

Level V: routine care that can be provided up to 4 hours after presentation (e.g., bruises, prescription refills, suture removal).

24. Are triage scoring methods precise?

Not exactly. Over- and undertriage are common problems in trauma systems.

25. Define over- and undertriage.

Overtriage occurs when minimally injured patients are triaged to a trauma center; undertriage occurs when severely injured patients are transported to a nontrauma center.

26. Which is worse: overtriage or undertriage?

Undertriage, which may result in preventable mortality or morbidity from delay of definitive care.

27. What is an acceptable undertriage rate for trauma systems?

Most trauma systems accept an undertriage rate of up to 10%. Each system must evaluate its triage criteria to provide the best quality of care to the community.

28. How are undertriaged patients transferred to the appropriate facility?

Through interfacility transfer agreements and protocols.

29. Who defines the interfacility transfer agreements?

Interfacility agreements should be made at a local or regional level. The trauma center should facilitate admission of patients who need a higher level of care than a community hospital is capable of providing.

30. What is an injury scoring system?

An objective system to measure severity of injury. Most authorities cite three injury scales: the Abbreviated Injury Scale (AIS), the Injury Severity Score (ISS), and the Trauma Score (TS).

31. How is the AIS score calculated?

The AIS divides the body into seven regions and uses a severity score from 1 to 6 for each injury. The score is calculated from the three most severely injured regions. A score of 1 indicates minor injury, whereas a score of 6 is fatal. Mortality increases as the AIS score increases.

32. Define the ISS.

The ISS score is defined as the sum of the squares of the highest AIS score in each of the graded body regions.

33. How is the TS calculated?

The TS is a prospective tool to determine survival probability. It combines the Glasgow Coma Scale (GCS) with respiratory and circulatory measurements to calculate a score between 1 and 12. The lower the score, the higher the mortality rate.

34. How are injured children evaluated?

The Pediatric Trauma Score (PTS) takes the special characteristics of pediatric patients into consideration. It is used as a prospective tool to determine survival probability in children.

35. Describe the TRISS method.

TRISS is the TS plotted against the ISS to calculate the probability of survival (PS).

36. What is the PS?

PS is a formula that considers patient age, severity of anatomic injury (ISS), and physiological status (TS) to determine statistically the probability of unexpected outcomes, positive or negative.

37. How is TRISS used?

As a method to compare trauma patient populations.

38. Why compare trauma populations?

To benchmark with like institutions of like size and patient population to trend outcomes.

39. How do trauma centers know whether they are "doing it right"?

Through quality management or performance improvement (PI) activities. PI provides a multidisciplinary approach to measure, evaluate, and improve the process and thus improve the outcome.

40. What activities are evaluated through the PI process?

Most PI activities focus on cost efficiency, resource utilization, and quality outcomes.

41. Describe the major goals of PI indicators.

- To improve patient care and work process
- To enhance productivity and provide professional development of nursing and allied health staff
- To identify opportunities and effective strategies for cost reduction as well as improvements that yield cost savings

42. How are quality PI indicators identified?

Indicators can be identified through regulatory agencies, professional groups, the healthcare institution, and/or the trauma department.

BIBLIOGRAPHY

1. Bureau of Health Services Resources, Division of Trauma and Emergency Medical Services: Model Trauma Care System Plan. Health Resources and Services Administration, U. S. Department of Health and Human Services, Rockville, MD, 1992.
2. Committee on Trauma, American College of Surgeons: Resources For Optimal Care of the Injured Patient: 1999. Chicago, American College of Surgeons, 1998.
3. Emergency Nurses Association: Course in Advanced Trauma Nursing: A Conceptual Approach. Park Ridge, IL, Emergency Nurses Association, 1995.
4. Furnival RA, Schunk JE: ABCs of scoring systems for pediatric trauma. Pediatr Emerg Care 15:215–223, 1999.
5. McQuillan KA, et al (eds): Trauma Nursing: From Resuscitation through Rehabilitation, 3rd ed. Philadelphia, Mosby, 2002.
6. Rutledge R, Osler T, Emery S, Kromhout-Schiro S: The end of Injury Severity Score (ISS) and the Trauma and Injury Severity Score (TRISS): ICISS, an International Classification of Diseases, ninth revision-based prediction tool, outperforms both ISS and TRISS as predictors of trauma patient survival, hospital charges, and hospital length of stay. J Trauma 44:41–49, 1998.
7. Sacco WJ, MacKenzie EJ, Champion HR, et al: Comparison of alternative methods for assessing injury severity based on anatomic descriptors. J Trauma 47:441–446, 1999.
8. Senkowski CK, McKenney MG: Trauma scoring systems: A review. J Am Coll Surg 189:491–503, 1999.

2. BIOMECHANICS AND MECHANISM OF INJURY

Richard L. Herm, RN, BSN, CEN, CNRN

1. Define biomechanics.
Biomechanics is the application of physics to injury research by examining how forces act on an object and how the object responds to these forces.

2. Define mechanism of injury.
Mechanism of injury refers to the methods by which different forms of energy from the environment are transferred to the victim of a traumatic event.

3. What are the five forms of energy that cause injury?
1. Mechanical/kinetic
2. Thermal
3. Chemical
4. Electrical
5. Radiant

4. What is deceleration force?
Deceleration force is the force that stops or decreases the velocity of a moving object or victim. It is dissipated on impact and must be absorbed around the impact site, including the victim. This energy causes blunt trauma.

5. What is acceleration force?
Acceleration force increases the amount of energy that is applied to a slower moving object, thus increasing its velocity. The greater the difference in velocity between the two objects, the greater the potential for injury.

6. Why is it important to know the mechanism of injury?
The mechanism of injury is a fundamental piece of information that helps to anticipate potential injuries and their severity. This information allows the members of the emergency department to better prepare themselves and the institution to care for the patient before arrival.

7. What are the two most common mechanisms of injury?
Blunt and penetrating trauma.

8. Name the mechanisms of injury that cause blunt trauma.
Blunt trauma results from deceleration forces that are transferred to the body during a motor vehicle crash involving cars, trucks, motorcycles, airplanes, motorized water craft, or other objects in motion. Acceleration forces also can cause blunt injury; for example, when a pedestrian, bicycle rider, or slower moving vehicle is struck by a faster moving vehicle. Other causes of blunt trauma include falls, especially from heights, and assaults with blunt objects.

9. What types of factors contribute to an occupant's injury pattern during a motor vehicle crash?
Factors that can contribute to an occupant's injury pattern include the use or nonuse of seat belts, availability of air bags, position of the victim in the vehicle, and whether it was a frontal, rear, lateral, angular, or rollover crash. The size and speed of the vehicle can also affect the pattern of injury.

10. What are the potential sites of injury in unrestrained occupants involved in a motor vehicle crash?

TYPE OF IMPACT	POTENTIAL INJURIES
Frontal	Head and neck
	Chest (heart, aorta, lungs, and rib or sternum fractures)
	Abdomen (liver, spleen, and intestines)
	Pelvis (ruptured bladder, torn urethra in males)
	Posterior hip dislocation
	Point-of-impact fractures to knee, femur, and ankle
	Lumbosacral spine (if only a lap belt is worn)
Lateral impact	Head and face, if victim is thrust forward
	Cervical spine
	Same-side shoulder and/or clavicle
	Lateral abdomen (liver of right-side occupant, spleen of left-side occupant)
	Diaphragm
Rear impact	Head and neck

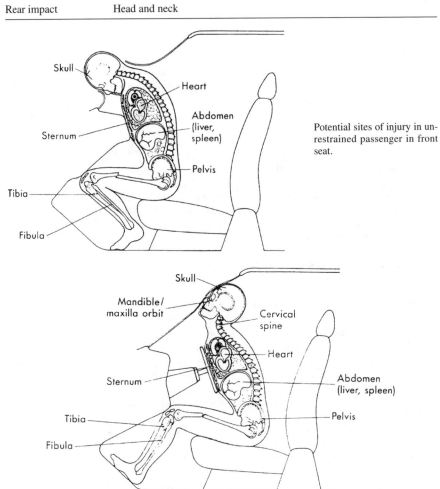

Potential sites of injury in unrestrained passenger in front seat.

Potential sites of injury in unrestrained driver.

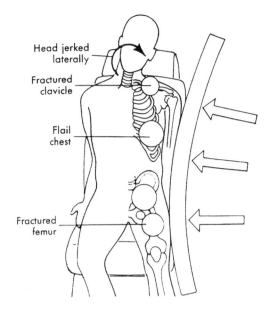

Potential sites of injury in lateral-impact collision. Note that injury is still possible in lateral crashes even with air bag inflation, because air bags were designed specifically for frontal crashes. However, injuries are usually fewer in lateral-impact crashes *with* air bag inflation than *without*.

Head jerked laterally

Fractured clavicle

Flail chest

Fractured femur

11. What mechanisms of injury are associated with penetrating trauma?

Mechanisms of injury that cause penetrating trauma include firearms, knives or instruments used for cutting or piercing, animals, machinery that can launch projectiles, high pressure equipment, and sharp objects or materials that can either become a weapon or impale the victim who falls on it.

12. Define cavitation.

Cavitation results from high-speed missiles or projectiles that penetrae tissue. As the energy from the projectile is dissipated in tissue, shock waves are created. These shock waves cause tissue compression and shear waves that create a temporary cavity larger than the size of the projectile. The properties of the pentrated tissue and the velocity of the projectile determine the degree and kind of tissue damage. The greater the velocity, the larger the cavitation.

13. Why is it important to know about cavitation?

It is important know about cavitation when caring for someone who has sustained a gunshot wound, because the volume of tissue destruction is usually much larger than is obvious from simply looking at the entrance and exit wounds. This hidden tissue destruction can lead to an increase in morbidity and mortality.

14. Which organ is most commonly injured by penetrating trauma to the abdomen?

The intestines.

15. Why is it helpful to know the angle at which a person was shot?

Knowing the angle at which the victim was shot can help determine whether more than one body compartment has been penetrated and what organs may be injured. This information facilitates rapid and appropriate treatment.

16. What injuries should be suspected in a person who falls or jumps from a height and lands on his or her feet?

Injuries from falling and landing on the feet may include fractures of the lower extremities and vertebral column. This type of injury is called **axial loading**. If the victim lands on his or her feet, then falls forward, bilateral wrist and knee fractures are also possible.

17. In what situations is a person exposed to both blunt and penetrating trauma?

The victim may be in a motorized vehicle and sustain a penetrating injury, such as a gunshot wound, that results in a crash, leading to the second mechanism of injury, blunt trauma. In another situation, victims caught in a fire may sustain a burn injury and have to jump from a height to save themselves. This scenario may lead to blunt injury from deceleration. A blast injury may cause blunt and penetrating trauma if the victim is hit by the blast shock wave and by a projectile that penetrates the skin. A victim who falls onto a protruding object and becomes impaled may sustain a deceleration injury along with the penetrating injury.

18. What mechanism of injury should be considered penetrating even though no guns, knives, or sharps objects are involved?

Contact with electrical energy may be considered a type of penetrating trauma. Once electricity enters the body, it can traverse through internal body structures and cause occult injuries that can be just as severe or worse than penetrating injury from a gun or knife.

19. What is the best initial treatment for chemical exposures to the skin?

Flush the exposed skin with a large amount of water.

20. What three types of collisions may occur during a motor vehicle crash?

1. The vehicle hits an object.
2. The occupants strike the inside of the vehicle.
3. The internal organs strike the inside of the body cavities that contain them.

For example, when a car hits a tree, the occupant's head may strike the windshield and the brain may strike the inside of the skull. The amount of energy transferred to the body of the victim ultimately determines the degree of injury.

21. Define compartment syndrome.

Compartment syndrome is a serious condition that can result from a crush injury or any injury in an area where there are tight fascial compartments. Increased pressure within the limited space of these compartments compromises the circulation and function of tissues within that space. Common locations include the anterior tibial and the deep posterior tibial compartments of the leg.

22. What is a coup-countrecoup injury in relation to head trauma?

Coup-countrecoup injury occurs during closed blunt head trauma. The head strikes an immovable object, such as a windshield, causing the brain to slam into the inside of the skull (the coup part of the injury). The countrecoup injury occurs as the inferior and frontal lobes are forced over the rough floor of the skull base, the middle and anterior fossae. These forces can cause direct neuronal damage and blood vessel tearing, resulting in intracranial, subdural, and/or subarachnoid hemorrhages.

23. How can an explosive blast cause tissue injury even if no projectile penetrates the body?

The explosive blast generates a shock wave with three components: positive phase, negative phase, and mass movement of air. These three phases cause massive changes in air pressure that can cause tissue damage. The **positive-pressure phase** is associated with velocities as high as 3000 m/sec, which decrease rapidly with increasing distance between the victim and the point of detonation. The **negative-pressure phase** follows the positive phase and lasts 10 times longer. The **mass movement of air phase** can actually cause tissue disruption, traumatic amputation, and evisceration. The most commonly injured tissues are those with tissue–air interfaces. Damage in the lung affects the alveolar wall, with resultant hemorrhage and edema. The abdominal organs sustain damage to the visceral wall, and the trauma may cause perforation.

24. What conditions other than compartment syndrome can result from a crush injury?

In addition to causing fractures, crush injuries can damage the underlying fascia. In some cases fascial injury can develop into necrotizing fasciitis, a condition that can cause rapid destruction of the subcutaneous tissue and deep fascia. Death is a common outcome.

BIBLIOGRAPHY

1. Campbell JE: Basic Trauma Life Support Advance Prehospital Care. Bowie, MD, Brady Communications, 1985.
2. Emergency Nurses Association: Trauma Nursing Core Course. Park Ridge, IL, Emergency Nurses Association, 2000.
3. Emergency Nurses Association: Course in Advanced Trauma Nursing: A Conceptual Approach. Park Ridge, IL, Emergency Nurses Association, 1995.
4. Neff JA, Kidd PS: Trauma Nursing: The Art and Science. St. Louis, Mosby, 1993.
5. Sheehy SB, Jimmerson CL: Manual of Critical Trauma Care: The First Hour, 2nd ed. St. Louis, Mosby, 1994.

3. STABILIZATION, TRANSFER, AND TRANSPORT

John J. Mason, RN, CEN, CFRN

1. What law governs the stabilization, transfer, and transport of trauma patients?

The Consolidated Omnibus Budget Reconciliation Act (COBRA) is the law requiring hospitals to conduct appropriate medical screening examinations for all patients presenting to the emergency department. The hospital is obligated to treat, stabilize, and, if necessary, appropriately transfer patients suffering from identified emergency conditions.

2. What is EMTALA?

EMTALA is the Emergency Medical Treatment and Labor Act. EMTALA requires hospitals and physicians that participate in Medicare to screen patients competently for emergency medical conditions, to stabilize emergent conditions, and to provide protected transfer. Hospitals and physicians that do not follow the requiremenents of EMTALA are subject to federal penalties for failure to provide appropriate emergency care.

3. Who makes the arrangements to transfer a trauma patient from one hospital to another? Who decides the mode of transport?

The sending physician is responsible for making the decision to transfer trauma patients. The sending physician must be in contact with the accepting physician. The accepting physician may offer the use of hospital-based services, if available, but ultimately the sending physician must decide the mode of transport. The sending physician should always get the name of the accepting physician.

4. How does a sending facility determine to which facility a trauma patient should be transferred?

The sending physician usually makes the final decision. This decision can be based on several factors, including written transfer agreements and type of specialty care available at the receiving facility (e.g., trauma center, burn, open-heart surgery, higher level of comprehensive care, pediatrics).

5. Discuss the different modes of transport.

Ground transport often is provided by local emergency medical service (EMS) personnel with training in basic and advanced life support (BLS, ALS). It may provide a quicker response time but most likely will result in an extended transport time. Another option is the critical care transport unit, a group of specially trained personnel often provided by the receiving facility. This mode may take longer for arrival, but it may be the only option available if weather conditions make other forms of transport uncertain.

Fixed-wing transport (Lear jet, Turbo-prop) is appropriate when extended distances must be covered to reach an appropriate facility. This mode of transport may require a longer period to arrange, because often it must be approved in advance by insurance companies. Fixed-wing transport is usually not appropriate for immediate trauma transfers.

Rotor-wing transport (helicopter) is the most rapid form of transport. Rotor-wing programs may be hospital-based or in out-based rural areas. Although there are many benefits of this form of transport, it can be uncertain because of maintenance schedules or weather conditions. Rotor-wing transport also provides a limited flight radius, which makes it inappropriate for long-distance transports.

6. What records are required at the time of transport?

Copies of all medical records relevant to the patient's care, as well as any radiology films (plain films, computed tomography scan, magnetic resonance imaging scan), should be sent with the patient. The physician's authorization and patient/family consent are also necessary for transport. Implied consent may be considered if no immediate family members are available. Documentation of the risks and benefits of transport also should be reviewed, ensuring that the benefits outweigh the risks. The effect of EMTALA laws also should be considered.

7. What communications should be made before the patient is transferred out of the facility?

The sending and receiving physicians must communicate verbally with one another. In addition, the nurse caring for the patient must telephone a report to the receiving facility. It is best to speak to either the charge nurse or the nurse who will receive the patient. This approach limits discrepancies in the transfer of care.

8. Who should accompany the trauma patient during transport?

Transport teams have different configurations based on the requirements of the patient. In the case of a trauma patient, the team most likely will include a registered nurse and a paramedic or respiratory therapist. The transport nurse should have a skilled background, ranging from the emergency department to intensive care. The team configuration can also vary depending on the amount of space in the transport vehicle. A ground unit or fixed-wing aircraft is usually capable of carrying extra transport team members and probably can accommodate family members. A helicopter, however, usually cannot accommodate more than two providers and the patient.

9. What should be assessed initially in trauma patients and then again during transport?

A primary survey should be completed for all trauma patients. This assessment consists of the ABCDs:

A = **A**irway. Ensure a patent airway. Assess the patient with simultaneous cervical spine immobilization to evaluate for trauma or tracheal deviation.

B = **B**reathing. Evaluate the patient's respiratory status, looking for flail segments, retractions, pneumothorax, respiratory distress, and anything that may require an intervention.

C = **C**irculation. Evaluate peripheral pulses, capillary refill, heart sounds, and blood pressure (either noninvasive or intra-arterial).

D = **D**isability (neurologic). A brief neurologic evaluation should consist of pupillary response, verbal response, and motor movement. A common evaluation tool is the Glasgow Coma Scale, which evaluates eye opening, verbal response, and motor response. Another tool is the AVPU, which relies on the patient's response to stimulus (**a**wake, **v**erbal, responds to **p**ain stimulus, or **u**nresponsive to painful stimulus).

10. What signs and symptoms indicate that a trauma patient is experiencing pain?

Patients express pain in many different ways. Regardless of whether or not the trauma patient is able to verbalize pain, it is important to establish baseline data. If the patient is unable to verbalize, physiologic indications of pain include tachypnea, tachycardia, hypotension, hypertension, and diaphoresis.

11. What treatments should be completed before and remain in place during transport?

The trauma patient should be fully immobilized with a long spine board, cervical collar, and head-blocks (unless the sending physician has cleared the cervical spine). The patient should have two large-bore intravenous lines that are patent, including blood tubing for infusing fluids or blood products. If there is any concern about the loss of the airway, the patient needs to be intubated; the endotracheal tube must be secured *before* transport. All identified fractures must be stabilized.

12. During fluid resuscitation, what important factors must trauma nurses consider?
- Monitor the patient's physiologic response to the resuscitation (vital signs).
- Monitor the patient's core body temperature, because most intravenous fluids are stored at room temperature and blood products are received cold. It is best to warm the intravenous fluids or blood with a warming device during infusion.

13. What methods are commonly used for warming the trauma patient?
Common methods include warm blankets, increasing room temperature, and warm intravenous fluids or blood products. Commercial devices include warming blankets and fluid warmers. The use of reflective blankets and head covers also helps to preserve body heat and to prevent additional heat loss, especially during transport.

14. What special considerations should be kept in mind during both fixed-wing and rotor-wing transport?
- Both the patient and the crew, particularly with rotor-wing transport, should use some form of hearing protection (e.g., helmet, headset, earplugs).
- Be aware of fumes from the engines, which produce carbon monoxide. During engine start-up or shut-down, keep the doors closed as long as possible. Carbon monoxide has a 300% higher affinity for hemoglobin than oxygen.
- Temperature is an important consideration for patients during transport. For every increase of 1000 feet, the temperature decreases by 3°F.
- Positioning during fixed-wing transport is important. In particular, gravitational forces can play an important role during fixed-wing transport. For example, a patient with a head injury should be placed head-first into the aircraft, whereas a patient with poor cardiac output should *not* be placed head-first in the aircraft during take-off.

15. What is the highest priority during transport?
Safety is the highest priority during transport. Safety factors include weather, traffic, and protection of the flight crew from a hostile environment. The goal is to go home at the end of the day.

16. How does weather factor into the transport decision for trauma patients?
Ground units are able to withstand rougher weather conditions in which visibility is decreased. With fixed-wing and rotor-wing transport, the pilots have the final decision. For example, when weather conditions make fixed-wing or rotor-wing transport unavailable, a ground unit may be able to transport the patient. The transport team, as a whole unit, should be involved in the decision, expressing any concerns before departure.

17. What does the transport team need to consider about intra-arterial pressure lines once a fixed-wing or rotor-wing aircraft reaches flying altitude?
According to Boyle's law, also known as the law of gaseous expansion, all invasive lines should be recalibrated or rezeroed once higher altitudes are reached. Air should be removed from all intravenous and intra-arterial pressure lines, because any air trapped within the fluid bags can alter infusion rates.

18. How often should patients be reassessed during transport?
Reassessment is often patient-specific. Depending on the transport time and patient stability, reassessments are done and documented in accordance with the transport team's preestablished protocol.

BIBLIOGRAPHY

1. Emergency Nurses Association: Trauma Nursing Core Course: Provider Manual, 4th ed. Park Ridge, IL, Emergency Nurses Association, 1995.
2. Frank G: EMTALA: An expert tells us what it's all about. J Emerg Nurs 27:65–67, 2001.
3. Holleran RS (ed): Flight Nursing: Principles and Practice, 2nd ed. St. Louis, Mosby. 1996.
4. National Flight Nurses Association: Flight Nursing Core Curriculum. Park Ridge, IL, National Flight Nurses Association, 1997.
5. Snyder A (ed): Certified Flight Registered Nurse Study Guide, 2nd ed. Park Ridge, IL, National Flight Nurses Association, 1996.
6. Wood J: eMedicine Journal, Vol. 2, No. 6, June 1, 2001,

II. Clinical Applications in Trauma Nursing Care

4. WEAPONS OF MASS DESTRUCTION AND BIOTERRORISM

Sharon Saunderson Cohen, RN, MSN, CEN, CCRN,
and Jeanne Eckes-Roper, RN, BSPA-HCA

1. Why are weapons of mass destruction (WMDs) a concern to the trauma nurse?

Terrorist or WMD events are usually related to traumatic injuries. The common dispersal device for WMD often is incendiary or explosive. Both methods of dispersal have the potential to cause a mass casualty incident.

2. Define terrorism.

The Department of Justice defines terrorism as a violent act or an act dangerous to human life in violation of the criminal laws of the United States to intimidate or coerce a government, civilian population, or any segment thereof in furtherance of political or social objectives.

3. Where does terrorism occur?

Terrorism can occur domestically (within the U.S.) or internationally.

4. What is considered a terrorist incident?

Terrorist incidents involving biologic, nuclear, incendiary, chemical, and environmental methods are considered technologically hazardous and are commonly described as weapons of mass destruction.

5. Define bioterrorism.

Bioterrorism is the deliberate use of microorganisms to cause disease with the intention of achieving a purpose or promoting a cause.

6. Define the acronym B-NICE.

WMDs include several types of incidents that may involve any of the following:

B = **B**iologic weapons
N = **N**uclear weapons
 I = **I**ncendiary weapons
C = **C**hemical weapons
E = **E**xplosives

7. Before beginning to care for a victim of a potential exposure to an unknown substance or agent, what types of harm to self must the nurse consider?

An easy way to remember potential harm or exposure is the acronym **TRACEM**:

T = **T**hermal exposure
R = **R**adiologic exposure
A = **A**sphyxiation
C = **C**hemical exposure
E = **E**tiologic exposure
M = **M**echanical harm

8. Give examples of TRACEM exposures.

Thermal: extreme heat or cold, such as smoldering clothing.

Radiologic: exposure to alpha, beta, or gamma rays (e.g., radiation from patient x-rays).

Asphyxiation: caused by lack of oxygen in the air. Common causes are gases (e.g., argon, carbon dioxide) and chemical vapors (emitted by the patient or burning clothing) in a confined space.

Chemical: harm posed by toxic or corrosive materials such as sulfurics, caustics (e.g., lye), and other chemicals (most often organophosphates).

Etiologic: exposure to disease-causing organisms (in blood and bodily fluids), often called bioterrorism. Organisms may be bacteria (anthrax), rickettsia (Q fever, typhus), viruses (smallpox, ebola), or toxins derived from living organisms (botulism).

Mechanical: the most typical form of trauma. Examples include gunshot wounds, falls, motor vehicle crashes, or even injury from bomb fragments or shrapnel.

9. The Centers for Disease Control and Prevention (CDC) have ranked most biologic agents into categories. What is the significance of category A for trauma nurses?

Category A is the highest priority to the CDC because the agents so classified have the highest potential for harm and weaponization. Category A agents can be easily disseminated or transmitted from person to person; cause high mortality rates, with the potential for major impact on public health; may cause public panic and social disruption; and require special action for public health preparedness.

10. Summarize the biologic characteristics of the six agents listed in category A.

AGENT	MICROBIOLOGY	RESERVOIR	INCUBATION
Anthrax	*Bacillus anthracis*, a spore-forming gram-positive rod	Livestock and wildlife Spores viable in soil for years	Average: 1–7 days Range: 1–60 days
Plague	*Yersinia pestis*, a gram-negative rod	Wild rodents	1–7 days (longer in immunocompromised hosts)
Smallpox	Variola virus, an orthopoxvirus	Only samples are contained within labs of government(s)	7–19 days
Botulism	Neurotoxins produced by the anaerobic gram-positive rod *Clostridium botulinum*	Spores, ubiquitous in soil	12–36 hours to several days
Tularemia	*Francisella tularensis*, a gram-negative rod	Wild animals (rabbits, beavers, various ticks)	Average: 5–10 days Range: 1–14 days
Hemorrhagic fever	Ebola and Marburg, filoviruses	Unknown Bats	Average: 5–10 days Range: 2–19 days

11. How are the six agents in category A transmitted?

Anthrax: inhalation and/or ingestion of spores, cutaneous contact with infected animal or spore through open skin.

Plague: bites from fleas from infected rodents.

Smallpox: inhalation, contact with skin lesions or secretions.

Botulism: inhalation or ingestion of spores.

Tularemia: tick bites, handling or eating insufficiently cooked meats, drinking contaminated water, inhalation of contaminated soil.

Hemorrhagic fever: contact with body fluid of infected person.

12. What diagnostic studies may be used for victims of category A diseases?

AGENT	DIAGNOSTIC STUDY
Anthrax	Widened mediastinum on chest x-ray
	Gram-positive bacilli in unspun blood smear, cerebrospinal fluid, nasal swab, sputum, or wound culture from cutaneous lesion
	Pathologic study showing hemorrhagic mediastinitis, hemorrhagic thoracic lymphadenitis, hemorrhagic meningitis
Plague	Sputum, blood, lymph node aspirate
	Gram-negative bacilli with bipolar (safety-pin) staining
	Pulmonary infiltrates or consolidation on chest x-ray
	Pathologic study showing lobular exudates, bacillary aggregation and areas of necrosis in pulmonary parenchyma
Smallpox	Vesicular or pustular fluid or scab in high concentrations seen under microscopy
	Growth of virus needed to definitive diagnosis
Botulism	Clinical diagnosis is foundation for early recognition; routine lab testing is unremarkable
	Electromyogram with normal nerve conduction velocity, normal sensory nerve function
	Serum or stool sample sent for testing
Tularemia	Small gram-negative coccobacilli in direct stain of respiratory secretions
	Peribronchial infiltrates leading to bronchopneumonia in one or more lobes on chest x-ray, often with pleural effusion and enlarged hilar nodes
	Target organs for acute suppurative necrosis followed by granulomatous reactions are lungs, lymph nodes, spleen, liver, and kidneys
Hemorrhagic fever	Enzyme-linked immunosorbent assay (ELISA), IgG or IgM, or viral antigen; viral isolation
	Often diagnosed post-mortem

13. What protective measures should a trauma nurse consider before coming into contact with a potentially infected or exposed patient?
- Specialized mask, such as the N/R 95 (for hazards such as pulmonary tuberculosis), P100 (for hazards such as hantavirus), or the powered air-purifying respirator (PAPR) with a full facepiece (even more protective)
- Disposable protective clothing with integral hood and booties
- Disposable nitrile or vinyl gloves
- Disposable rubber shoe coverings with ridged soles

Additional equipment may or may not be necessary, depending on the agent and exposure.

14. What are the three levels of personal protective equipment (PPE)?

Level A: The level of protective equipment for situations in which the material is considered acutely vapor-toxic to the skin and hazards are unknown. Equipment includes full encapsulation, airtight chemical suit with self-contained breathing apparatus (SCBA), or supplied air breathing apparatus (SABA).

Level B: The level of protective equipment for situations in which the environment is not considered acutely vapor-toxic to skin but may cause respiratory effects. Equipment includes chemical splash suit or full coverage, non–air-tight chemical suit with SCBA or SABA.

Level C: The level of protective equipment required to prevent respiratory exposure but not to exclude possible skin contact. Equipment includes chemical splash suit with cartridge respirator.

Level D: The level of protective equipment required when the atmosphere contains no known hazard and when splashes, immersions, inhalation, or contact with hazardous levels of any chemical is precluded. Equipment includes work uniform such as coveralls, boots, leather gloves, and hard hat.

15. What chemical agents may be involved in a terroristic event?
Chemical agents are categorized as follows:
- Nerve agents (tabun, organophosphates, soman, sarin gas)
- Vesicants (mustard gas, lewisite)
- Cyanides or blood agents (hydrogen cyanide, cyanogen chloride)
- Pulmonary or choking agents (chlorine, phosgene)
- Irritants (tear gas, Mace, pepper spray)

16. What are other weapons of mass destruction?
Explosives may be used by themselves or as a means of spreading biologic, chemical, or nuclear agents. Another weapon may be an **incendiary device** (fire, Molotov cocktail).

17. List in proper sequence the treatment procedures that should be followed according to local protocols.
1. Gross decontamination (done at scene by hazmat teams; level A equipment is needed)
2. Patient management (begins at scene)
3. Transport to appropriate medical facility
4. Definitive care (at hospital/trauma center; may begin with fine decontamination)

18. What is gross decontamination?
Gross decontamination is the initial removal of a contaminating substance/agent that may pose a health threat to the patient or health care team. Gross decontamination includes removal of all contaminated clothing and jewelry and external cleansing of skin surfaces.

19. What is fine decontamination?
Fine decontamination is the meticulous decontamination of a patient's "nooks and crannies" (e.g., nasal passages, ears, other orifices).

20. By what mechansims do organophosphates do harm?
Organophosphates are nerve agents that inhibit acetylcholinesterase. As a result, the nerve impulses never rest and continue to fire, resulting in convulsions and other uncontrolled muscle reactions.

21. How common are organophosphates?
Organophosphates are found in many household insecticidal sprays and fertilizers. They are also found commercially in more concentrated forms that can kill within minutes of exposure.

22. What is off-gassing?
Gases may remain on the clothing of an exposed victim and cause contamination in the surrounding area(s) or of health care personnel.

23. What are the signs and symptoms of exposure to a nerve agent?
The signs and symptoms of exposure to a nerve agent can be remembered by the acronym **SLUDGEM**:
S = **S**alivation
L = **L**acrimation
U = **U**rination
D = **D**efecation
G = **G**astric distress
E = **E**mesis
M = **M**iosis

24. What is the usual treatment for a trauma patient exposed to a nerve agent?

In addition to interventions of advanced trauma life support (ATLS), the trauma nurse must attempt to reverse the effects of the nerve agent with atropine (an anticholinergic), pralidoxime chloride (an oxime), and diazepam (an anticonvulsant). This treatment should be delivered in a well-ventilated area (possibly outside the trauma center or emergency department) and simultaneously with decontamination.

25. If a WMD event is suspected, whom should the trauma nurse notify?

The nurse should notify local EMS (prehospital providers) hazardous material response teams, local infection control personnel, local and state health departments, and local, state, and federal law enforcement officials.

26. Which law enforcement agency has jurisdiction over any act of WMD in the United States?

The Federal Bureau of Investigation (FBI) has ultimate authority over any aspect of a WMD event in the U.S. Any WMD act is a federal offense. Local law enforcement assists in the investigation and contacts the FBI.

27. What is a unified incident command? How important is it?

Incident command is the structured form of on-scene crisis management that ensures that all participating agencies are effectively communicating within the designated command structure. A strong incident command fosters scene and personnel safety.

28. What are the three components of incident command?

1. Establishing and updating priorities, such as life safety, incident stabilization, property and environmental conservation, and investigation of cause and origin.

2. Continual assessment of both the present situation and the predicted behavior of the incident and patient population under treatment.

3. Establishing and updating incident priorities, with a focus on what needs to be done, how it will be done, and when and who will do it.

29. Do emergency departments and trauma centers use the incident command structure?

Any large-scale incident that exceeds the normal flow of an area of a hospital should use the incident command structure to evaluate, plan, and act in a timely fashion. The ultimate goal is to treat incoming patients while fostering health care worker safety. A hospital-based incident commander should be in contact with the on-scene incident commander for complete assessment of the incident.

30. What are NBCs?

NBCs are methods used as weapons of mass destruction:

N = Nuclear
B = Biologic
C = Chemical

31. Explosives are often used as dispersal agents in WMD. What are the three primary effects produced by explosives when they are detonated?

1. **Blast pressure** occurs in two phases. First, positive blast pressure moves rapidly away from the explosion center (ground zero) because of the expansion caused by the release of energy. After the positive-pressure phase, a vacuum is created at the explosion site. This vacuum creates a negative pressure, which moves toward the original center of the detonation at hurricane speed. It is less sudden but lasts approximately three times as long as the positive-pressure wave.

2. **Fragmentation** occurs when the explosive device propels fragments at high speed for long distances. This phase accounts for many of the injuries that present to the hospital as well as many of the casualties.

3. **Thermal effects** are also called incendiary effects. Heat produced by the detonation of either high or low explosives varies according to the ingredient materials. High explosives generate greater temperatures than low explosives, but the thermal effects from low explosives have a longer duration than those of high explosives.

32. Why is postevent management important?
Incident evaluation and management of critical incident stress are essential to the well-being of the involved personnel.

33. What is a critical incident?
A critical incident is any event that has sufficient power to overwhelm the normal coping strategies of the health care team members, creating the potential for interference with their ability to function.

34. Give examples of critical incidents.
• Traumatic death of a child.
• Disasters and/or mass casualty incidents (MCIs)
• Line-of-duty deaths or serious injuries to peers or other emergency workers (EMS/law enforcement)
• Events that attract excessive media attention
• Incidents associated with unusual circumstances and/or distressing sights, sounds, or smells
• Exposure to WMD events or substances/agents that may threaten the well-being of self or family

35. Are all personnel affected by critical incidents?
No. Every person responds differently, based on individual mental health and coping strategies. However, unless the critical incident stress is lessened, posttraumatic stress disorder (PTSD) may develop as a debilitating chronic condition.

36. Identify the signs and symptoms of stress.

Physical	Cognitive
Fatigue	Confusion
Nausea	Intrusive images
Muscle twitching	Nightmares
Chest pain	Cognitive deficits in:
Dyspnea	• Decision-making
Elevated blood pressure	• Concentration
Tachycardia	• Memory
Thirst	• Problem-solving
Headaches	• Abstract thinking
Visual difficulties	
Dizziness	
Emotional	
Anxiety	Loss of emotional control
Guilt	Depression
Grief	Apprehension
Denial	Intense anger
Fear	Irritability
Uncertainty	Agitation

Behavioral

Withdrawal	Pacing
Emotional outbursts	Nonspecific bodily complaints
Suspiciousness	Change in sexual functioning
Alcohol consumption	Changes in activity and speech
Inability to rest	

37. How long can symptoms of stress last?

Reactions to a stressful incident may occur quickly, from within a few minutes to hours, days, weeks, or even months after the event. These reactions may last an indefinite length of time.

38. Define critical incident stress management (CISM)?

CISM provides health care team members the opportunity to deal with their emotions and return to a productive level of functioning.

39. How does the process of CISM work?

CISM may include the use of defusing and/or debriefing techniques. **Defusing** sessions are usually short and done on a relatively informal basis at the time or near the conclusion of the incident. They allow the involved personnel to ventilate their feelings about the incident. **Debriefings** are more structured and organized sessions conducted within 24–72 hours of the incident with the objective of providing the health care team members the opportunity to deal with their emotions.

40. Who conducts the debriefings? Who is on the team?

Critical incident stress teams are a partnership among mental health professionals, emergency service workers, and medical/nursing health care providers who are interested in preventing and mitigating the negative impact of stress on themselves and their coworkers.

41. What steps are involved in the debriefing process?

There are seven steps to a debriefing:

1. **Initial phase:** Introductions are made, and the ground rules for the session are clearly stated.

2. **Fact phase:** Members of the health care team discuss their role in the event and describe their participation in what was done, seen, and heard.

3. **Thought phase:** Participants who are willing to speak share what they felt during the incident and how they personalized it.

4. **Reaction phase:** Each paticipant is allowed to share and describe personal reactions to the worst part of the event in a safe environment.

5. **Symptom phase:** Participants describe any symptoms that they may have experienced as a result of the incident or since the time of the incident.

6. **Teaching phase:** Team members provide stress-reducing strategies and/or methods to support one another during a crisis.

7. **Re-entry phase:** The group has the opportunity to ask additional questions.

42. Is CISM debriefing mandatory?

All personnel involved in a critical incident should be required to attend the debriefing session, but individual participation is voluntary.

43. By what mechanisms is a CISM team called out?

Institutional protocols should be developed to determine when and where a CISM team may respond. Protocols should stipulate that any team member at any level of service may initiate a call-out for the CISM team. Protocols should be available and accessible at all times.

BIBLIOGRAPHY

1. Emergency Nurses Association: Crisis intervention. In Emergency Nursing Pediatric Course (Instructor) Manual. Park Ridge, IL, Emergency Nurses Association, 1993, pp 209–223.
2. Mitchell JT, Bray GP: Emergency Services Stress. Englewood Cliffs, NJ, RJ Brady/Prentice Hall, 1990.
3. Reese JT, Horn JM, Dunning C: Critical Incidents in Policing Revised. Washington, DC, Federal Bureau of Investigation, 1991.

Websites
http://www.apic.org
http://www.bt.cdc.gov
http://www.cdc.gov/ncidod/diseases/bioterr.htm
http://www.cdc.gov/ncidod/dbmd/anthrax.htm
http://www.cdc.gov/ncidod/diseases/foodborn/botu.htm
http://www.cdc.gov/ncidod/srp/drugservice/immuodrugs.htm
http://www.chemdef.apgea.army.mil/
http://www.fbi.gov/lab/bomsum/eubdc.htm
http://www.fema.gov
http://mrmc-www.army.mil/
http://www.nbc-med.org
http://www.nbc-ed.org/SiteContent/HomePage /WhatsNew/anthraxinfo/ Anthraxinfo3.htm
http://www.defenselink.mil/specials/Anthrax/anth.htm
http://www.hopkins-id.edu/bioterr/bioterr_1.html
http://www.who.int/emc-documents/zoonoses/docs/whoemczdi986.html
http://www.hopkins-biodefense.org
http://www.usamriid.army.mil/html/Home/home.asp
http://www.state.gov/www/global/terrorism

5. FORENSICS IN TRAUMA NURSING

Jeanne Eckes-Roper, RN, BSPA-HCA

1. Define forensic and forensic pathology.

Forensic means pertaining to the law. **Forensic pathology** is a subspecialty concerned with the investigation of death.

2. How do the fields of trauma nursing and forensics intersect?

Trauma nurses have long provided optimal care to trauma patients. Practitioners of trauma care must protect the patient's legal, civil, and human rights through the proper recognition, collection, and preservation of evidence in addition to the reporting of suspected forensic cases.

3. What is clinical forensic practice?

Clinical forensics is a specialty concerned primarily with the survivor of violent crimes or liability-related trauma.

4. When do nurses apply forensic principles during the care of the trauma patient?

Every day. Whenever care is provided to a trauma victim, the nurse should consider the art of forensics. Survivors of trauma include all victims of violence, motor vehicle/pedestrian crashes, burns, occupation-related injuries, gunshot and stab wounds, sexual battery, domestic violence (infant/child, spousal, and geriatric abuse), and suicide attempts.

5. Define forensic nursing.

Forensic nursing is the application of nursing science with the biopsychosocial education of the registered nurse in the scientific investigation and treatment of trauma and/or death of victims and perpetrators of violence, criminal activity, and traumatic incidents.

6. How do forensic nurses play a role in the investigation of death?

Forensic nurses are used to investigate death because of their nursing education. Nurses bring empathy and compassion as well as excellent observational, clinical, and communication skills to the investigation of death.

7. Define physical evidence.

Physical evidence is defined as any quantity of matter, material, or condition in a solid, liquid, or gaseous state that may be used to determine and/or support the facts in an investigation.

8. How does physical evidence help the investigator?

Physical evidence can accomplish any or all of the following:
- Link a victim to a crime
- Link a victim or subject to a crime scene
- Identify an assailant
- Establish an element of the crime
- Corroborate or disprove an alibi

9. Describe the purpose of evidence.

The purpose of evidence is to establish the facts of the crime:
- That a crime has been committed
- That a certain person has committed the crime
- The modus operandi (MO) of the crime

25

10. When should evidence be collected?
Whenever crashes or unintentional injury cases, traumatic injury cases, or suspicious deaths occur.

11. List examples of crashes and unintentional injury.
- Motor vehicle crashes
- Motorcycle/moped crashes
- Bicycle crashes
- Pedestrian incidents

12. List examples of traumatic injury cases.
- Gunshot and stab wounds
- Assaults
- Falls
- Burns

13. Define suspicious death.
A suspicious death is any unexplained death. Any death that occurs within 24 hours of admission to the hospital and all trauma resuscitation/emergency department deaths are considered suspicious.

14. What is a medicolegal case?
Any medical case with legal implications. All of the above cases fall into this category.

15. What role does the forensic nurse have in the collection and preservation of evidence?
It is the forensic nurse's responsibility to maintain the integrity of the evidence and the chain of custody until an investigating agency, law enforcement agency, and/or the medical examiner's office comes to claim the evidence.

16. What role does the trauma nurse have in the collection and preservation of evidence?
The trauma nurse is part of the initial team caring for the critically injured patient and may be the first person to come in contact with evidence.

17. Define chain of custody.
Chain of custody refers to the identity of the person or persons having control over evidentiary material or personal property. Each person having contact with evidence has a role in maintaining its integrity. Each person in possession of or having contact with evidence must be clearly identified for the courts.

18. Why is the chain of custody important?
The chain maintains integrity of the evidence and protects admissibility in court.

19. Where does the chain of custody begin?
With the first person who collects evidence. The person may be a member of the health care team, ranging from prehospital providers in the field to hospital staff, including but not limited to nurses, technicians, and physicians.

20. Can the confines of a hospital be considered a crime scene?
Yes. Sometimes critical evidence is lost as the medical team stabilizes and treats the patient. Often unstable patients are rapidly transported to the trauma center or emergency department for stabilization and treatment. Because medical treatment is the priority, evidence is overlooked or destroyed during the provision of medical care.

21. Why is evidence lost?

Most often evidence goes unrecognized. Examples of lost evidence include the following:
• Holes in clothing created by bullets from a gun are often cut through.
• Paint chips from a car that struck a patient are often brushed off clothing.
• Clothing that is cut off the patient and thrown on the floor can contaminate evidence.

22. How is evidence identified?

All articles of clothing and tissue can be used as evidence. Law enforcement officials investigating the traumatic incident or crime will determine what is and can be evidence. The trauma nurse must understand what can be identified as evidence and communicate with law enforcement officials.

23. How is evidence classified?

Physical evidence: any tangible article that tends to prove or disprove a point in question. It may be used to reconstruct a crime, identify participants, and/or confirm or discredit an alibi.

Trace evidence: hair, fibers, clothing, bullets/projectiles, foreign objects, and paint chips.

Transient (conditional) evidence: temporary in nature (e.g., odor, temperature, smoke, indentations, imprints from fire and light).

Patterned evidence: produced by physical contact between persons or objects (e.g., blood splatter, glass fractures, fire burn patterns, tire marks, projectile/trajectory patterns).

24. How is evidence used in defining a crime?

Evidence is used for the recognition, identification, classification, individualization, or reconstruction of events relating to a crime or potential crime. Evidence connects the person to a crime or potential crime. It may be the link between person, action, and outcome of the event.

25. Who identifies that evidence is present?

Any health care team member is capable of identifying forensic evidence. The investigating law enforcement agency should be notified if the presence of evidence is suspected.

26. How can evidence be protected during provision of care to the patient?

Use care when removing articles of clothing that may contain trace evidence. Do not throw clothing on the floor. Place all items in "breathable" paper bags. If the patient is thought to have fired or handled a weapon, place clean paper bags over the hands until tests for gunshot residue can be performed by the crime scene technicians.

27. Why place evidence in paper bags rather than plastic bags?

Plastic degrades evidence quickly, thereby limiting its value.

28. What evidence is considered to be the most accurate evidence available?

DNA evidence. It is as individual as a fingerprint.

29. What is the best method to obtain DNA evidence?

Crime labs do not need or want blood samples for DNA testing. Buccal swabs provide the best specimen. DNA can be retrieved from any area where saliva from the suspect may have been transferred, such as bite marks, breasts, neck, and skin.

30. How is DNA matched?

Through the Combined DNA Index System (CODIS).

31. What is CODIS?

Operated by the Federal Bureau of Investigation (FBI), this databank allows crime laboratories to store and match DNA records. It consists of four indices of DNA records:

1. Forensic index
2. Convicted offender index
3. Missing person index
3. Population file (anonymous DNA profiles)

32. What evidence is recognized by the courts?
1. **Direct evidence**, such as eye witness accounts, witness statement, or dying declaration.
2. **Circumstantial evidence**, such as physical evidence or statements that establish circumstances from which one can infer other facts at issue.
3. **Real evidence**, such as physical or tangible objects that may prove or disprove a statement in question. Real evidence may be direct or circumstantial.

33. How should evidence be documented?
Evidence can be documented by handwritten notes, sketches and drawings, photographs, audiotape, and videotape.

34. How are gunshot wounds evaluated for evidentiary value?
Gunshot wounds should be inspected for size, shape, characteristics, determination of distance, powder stippling, and contact wounds.

35. What is powder stippling?
The soot (powder burning/blackening) deposited on the wound margins by the projectile.

36. Describe the extent or forms of tissue damage caused by bullets from firearms.
1. Dissipation of the missile's kinetic energy in tissues ($K\Sigma \approx MV^2$)
2. Production of secondary missiles
3. Cavitation

37. Define cavitation.
A temporary cavity that refers to a localized area of blunt trauma along the projectile path; a stretch phenomenon.

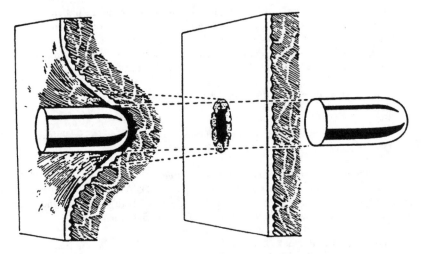

As a bullet penetrates the skin, the skin is pressed inward, stretched, and perforated in the stretched condition, after which it returns to its original position. The entry opening is smaller than the diameter of the bullet. Immediately around the opening is the contusion ring. The bullet rubs against this part of the skin and scrapes off the external layer of epithelial cells. (From Svensson A, et al: Techniques of Crime Investigation. New York, Elsevier Science, 1981, with permission.)

38. Identify the most common firearm in the United States that is associated with traumatic injuries.

The handgun is the most commonly used firearm in both homicides and suicides in the United States. Handguns are low-velocity, low-energy weapons with muzzle velocities below 1400 ft/sec.

39. List the four categories of wounds created by firearms.

Wounds are divided into four categories, depending on the distance from muzzle to target: contact, near-contact, intermediate, and distant.

40. What is a contact wound?

The muzzle of the gun is in hard, loose, or angled contact with the body. Loose contact results in deposition of a wider zone of soot around the entrance. Angled contact produces an oval-shaped zone of soot.

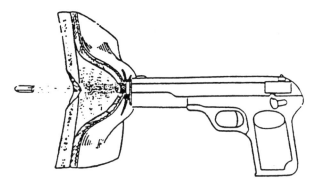

With a contact shot, the weapon is pressed against the head or the body. The gases from the explosion expand between the skin and the bone, producing a bursting effect and a ragged entrance wound. (From Svensson A, et al: Techniques of Crime Investigation. New York, Elsevier Science, 1981, with permission.)

41. Describe the appearance of a contact wound.

All contact wounds exhibit scorching of the wound edges and deposition of soot (powder burning/blackening) on the wound margins. In addition, soot and powder particles are driven into the wound tract. Some contact wounds may show a muzzle impression secondary to blowback of the skin caused by the discharged gases.

42. How do contact wounds over bone and over clothing differ?

Contact wounds over bone may have the following characteristics:
- A stellate wound at the entrance point is often produced by subcutaneous expansion of the powder gases between the skin and the bone.
- Soot is deposited around the entrance in the bone.

Contact wounds over clothing may have the following characteristics:
- Clothing absorbs the soot and powder elements.
- Clothing may be driven into the wound tract.
- Powder grains and soot are found in the wound tract.

43. Describe near-contact wounds.

Near-contact wounds lie in a gray zone between contact and intermediate-range wounds. The muzzle of the weapon is not in contact with the skin. The entrance wound is surrounded by a wide zone of powder soot overlying seared, blackened skin. Soot in the seared zone is baked into the skin and cannot be wiped away.

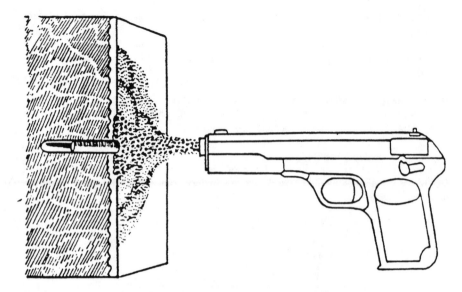

In a near-contact shot, both incompletely burned powder grains and smoke deposits are found in the zone of blackening. The powder grains are concentrated immediately around the entrance hole. (From Svensson A, et al: Techniques of Crime Investigation. New York, Elsevier Science, 1981, with permission.)

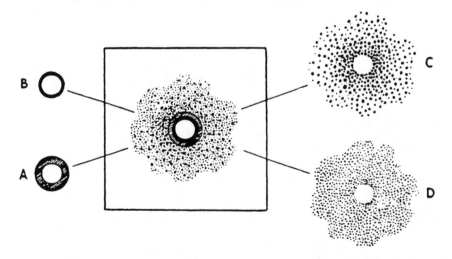

Marks that may be found around the entry opening of a bullet in a near-contact shot. *A,* Contusion ring; *B,* smudge ring; *C,* grains of powder; and *D,* deposit of powder residue. (From Svensson A, et al: Techniques of Crime Investigation. New York, Elsevier Science, 1981, with permission.)

44. Describe intermediate-range gunshot wounds.
- The muzzle of the weapon is held away from the body at the time of discharge.
- Powder grains produce "powder tattooing" of the skin. The powder grains cannot be wiped away.
- Powder tattoo marks are punctate lesions of the skin, reddish-brown to orange-red, surrounding the entrance of the wound.

- Powder tattooing is an antemortem sign.
- Soot (powder blackening) is present on close-up gunshot wounds (out to a maximum of 12 inches for handguns).
- The size and density of the powder tattoo pattern can be used to determine the range. Powder tattooing from rifles and shotguns is less dense than tattooing from handguns.
- Hair and clothing may interfere somewhat with powder tattooing. All clothing should be examined.

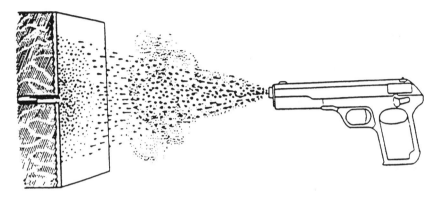

In intermediate-range shots, unburned powder grains but no smoke deposits are found in the zone of blackening. (From Svensson A, et al: Techniques of Crime Investigation. New York, Elsevier Science, 1981, with permission.)

45. Describe a distant gunshot wound.
- No soot or tattooing is present.
- The only marks on the target are produced by the mechanical action of the bullet in perforating the skin.
- The exact range of fire cannot be determined.
- The entrance wound can be determined from the exit wound.

46. How are entrance and exit wounds over skin determined?
Entrance wounds
- A reddish zone of abraded skin (called the abrasion ring) results from scraping of the bullet against the margin of the bullet hole as it perforates the skin. This rim of flattened, abraded epidermis surrounds the entrance hole.
- An abrasion ring is present in contact, close-up, and distant gunshot wounds.
- Except for contact wounds over bone (see question 47), entrance wounds tend to be small, circular or oval, and regular.
- Symmetrical abrasion rings suggest a head-on shot, whereas concentric rings indicate an angled shot.

Exit wounds
- Exit wounds usually are larger and more irregular than entrance wounds as a result of bullet tumble or yaw and bullet deformation.
- Usually no abrasion ring is present.
- The exit wound may have a stellate, crescent, circular, or completely irregular shape.

47. How are entrance and exit wounds over bone determined?
Entrance wounds usually have a stellate or cruciform appearance. The hole is beveled inward.

Exit wounds are beveled or cratered. The hole is beveled outward.

48. What other characteristics of gunshot wounds are important?

    1. X-ray distortion does not allow the caliber of the bullet to be identified in the body.

    2. Because of its elasticity, the caliber of a bullet cannot be identified by the entrance hole in the skin.

    3. The trajectory of the bullet through the body depends on the following factors:
- Position of the body
- Position of the assailant
- Angle at which the weapon was held

49. How do shotgun wounds differ from handgun wounds?

Shotguns have a smooth bore; although they can fire a single projectile, they usually are used to fire multiple pellets. Barrel lengths in shotguns range from 18 to 36 inches; the usual lengths are 26, 28, and 30 inches. A shotgun shell can contain several hundred pellets or one large slug. A wad or wads of paper or plastic may lie between the pellets. A shotgun wound is usually larger in diameter and causes more soft tissue damage than a wound created by a handgun.

50. Describe the characteristics of stab wounds.

    1. The shape and measurement of the wound match the knife.

    2. Physical characteristics of the knife and other instruments are observed on the wound (e.g., jagged pattern vs. smooth cut).

    3. The location of the wound (i.e., right vs. left side, front vs. back) may help to identify defense wounds.

51. What laboratory tests may be considered in forensics?

- **Blood alcohol concentration** (BAC). When BAC is determined, the technician should note whether the specimen was obtained from law enforcement officers or hospital personnel. This distinction has a significant impact in court because of the medical procedures and timing associated with hospital-drawn specimens.
- **Carbon monoxide levels** assist in the identification of the source (e.g., automobile, hibachi, air conditioning).
- **DNA analysis** assists in the identification of the individual source of the specimen.

52. What statements made by a patient are admissible in court?

    1. Statements made with the belief of impending death ("dying declaration")

    2. Statements against interest (admission or confession)

    3. Statements made for the purposes of medical diagnosis or treatment

    4. Statements of existing emotional or physical condition (state of mind)

53. Define dying declaration.

A statement made at a time when a person believes that he or she is dying about the circumstances and events that led to his or her present condition.

54. Does the patient have to die for a dying declaration to be valid and used in court?

No. The patient only needs to believe that he or she is dying.

55. What is an admission or confession?

Any statement made by a suspect against his or her interest.

56. Describe a statement made for purposes of medical diagnosis or treatment.

A statement made in conversation to a health care professional in the discharge of his or her duties can equate to a confession. Such statements become important in cases of driving under the influence of alcohol and domestic violence cases, in which a drug or alcohol level may be in question. For example, the patient may state that he or she has been drinking or ingesting drugs.

57. What is meant by statements of existing emotional or mental condition?
The patient's responsiveness to medical questions and treatment that can aid in determining the intent, plan, motive, or design of an event.

58. If evidence is documented and statements are taken during medical treatment, will the practitioner be subpoenaed to appear in court?
Not in all cases. Sometimes a clarification for the state attorney is all that is warranted.

59. Does the practitioner have an obligation to go to court?
If a subpoena is issued, the practitioner has an obligation to respond. Forensic nurses often testify in court to provide expert testimony in areas dealing with questionable death investigation processes, adequacy of service delivery, and specialized diagnoses of specific conditions related to nursing. Local laws and institutional policies should be valuable resources.

60. Define sexual battery.
Sexual battery or rape is defined as oral, anal, and/or vaginal penetration of another person or contact with a sexual organ of another person without consent. Sexual battery also includes anal or vaginal penetration with an object or body part other than sexual organs (e.g., fingers, bottles). Medical procedures are not considered sexual battery provided that they are performed by a bona fide medical practitioner for medical purposes (after appropriate consent is obtained).

61. How are forensic practice principles applicable to sexual assault victims?
Sexual assault cases require expertise and knowledge about legal and ethical responsibilities, physical examination and interviewing techniques, and evidence collection practices.

62. What is a sexual assault nurse examiner (SANE)?
A nurse who conducts an assessment and physical examination of victims of sexual battery is called a SANE nurse examiner. SANE nurses are experts in evidence collection and often are expected to testify in court about their investigative findings.

63. Where do SANE nurses practice?
SANE nurses may practice in a rape crisis center, emergency department, or trauma center. Some are independent contractors.

64. How common are child abuse and neglect? What are the general characteristics of abused children?
- 13.9 per 1000 children are victims of abuse or neglect, and 42.0 per 1000 are harmed or endangered.
- Mortality rate: > 2000 per year (> 75% of deaths are in children < 3 years old)
- Gender: female, 52%; male, 48%
- Ethnicity: white, 67%; African-American, 27%; Hispanic, 13%

65. Define abuse and neglect.
Abuse
- A willful or threatened act that results in physical, mental, or sexual injury
- Harm that causes or is likely to cause significant impairment of a child's physical, mental, or emotional health
- Includes acts of omission
Neglect
- Deprivation of necessary food, clothing, shelter, or medical care
- Allowing a child to live in an environment that causes significant impairment of physical, mental, or emotional health or places the child in danger

• Includes willful acts that result in sprains, cartilage damage, bone or skull fracture, brain or spinal damage, intercranial hemorrhage, asphyxiation, drowning, burns, lacerations, bites, internal injuries, disfigurement, and impairment of body part or function
• Giving a child alcohol, drugs, or poisons that result in sickness or affect behavior

66. When should child abuse or neglect be suspected?
Abuse or neglect is often suspected when the child's injuries and the history provided by a caregiver do not match. Abuse or neglect is also suspected in the presence of signs of previous abuse (old, healing fractures or perhaps bruises/contusions in various stages of healing).

67. Can a child be detained without caregiver consent if abuse or neglect is suspected?
Absolutely. A report must be made whenever there is reasonable suspicion that a child has been abused, abandoned, or neglected.

68. When is abuse not abuse?
Sometimes cultural rituals and religious health practices are mistaken for abuse situations. Careful investigations should be undertaken. Coining and cupping can be confused with burns and bruises. Mongolian spots also can be confused with bruises.

69. Discuss the forensic aspects of elder abuse.
• Passive/active neglect: the caretaker is well intentioned but unable to meet the elder's needs; the caretaker intentionally over- or undermedicates or withholds life necessities.
• Physical abuse: battery of an elder.
• Psychological abuse: intimidating verbal contact, profanity, threats, belittling, and instilling fear of being put in a nursing home.
• Financial abuse: the caretaker squanders the elder's funds or property or refuses to expend funds for necessities. Fraud or embezzlement also may be involved.

70. List the common areas of forensic nursing.
Death investigators
Trauma and emergency department nurses
Correctional nurse specialists
Forensic psychiatric nurses
Legal nurse consultants
Forensic geriatric specialists
Nurse attorneys
Sexual assault nurse examiners

71. Define forensic nurse specialist.
A forensic nurse specialist is a registered nurse who provides direct services to individual clients; consultation services to nursing, medical, and law-related agencies; or expert court testimony in areas dealing with questionable death investigation processes, adequacy of service delivery, and specialized diagnoses of specific conditions related to nursing. Several states now offer courses specializing in forensic nursing.

72. Is forensic nursing a recognized nursing specialty?
Yes. Forensic nursing received formal recognition in 1991 at the Annual Meeting of the American Academy of Forensic Sciences. In 1992 the discipline of forensic nursing was formally organized and is now represented by a nursing specialty association.

73. What is this specialty association?
The International Association of Forensic Nurses (IAFN) was established in Minneapolis, Minnesota, on August 12, 1992.

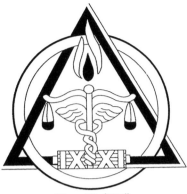

"Beyond Tradition"

Emblem of the International Association of Forensic Nurses. (Reprinted with permission of the International Association of Forensic Nurses.)

74. Summarize the mission statement of the IAFN.
Its primary objective is to ensure that nurses develop a role that will have a great impact on the future of both forensic science and health care professions. Forensic nursing is seen as an important part of the solution to the nation's most pressing problem: violence.

BIBLIOGRAPHY

1. Besant-Matthews P: Keys to the Crime: Evidence Collection in Trauma. Lewisville, TX, Barbara Clark Mims Associates, 1991.
2. DiMaio VJM: Gunshot Wounds: Practical Aspects of Firearms, Ballistics, and Forensic Techniques. Boca Raton, FL, CRC Press, 1985.
3. Goll-McGee B: The role of the clinical forensic nurse in critical care. Crit Care Nurs Q 22:8–18, 1999.
4. Hobbs CJ, et al: Child Abuse and Neglect: A Clinician's Handbook. London, Harcourt Brace, 1999.
5. Lynch VA: Injuries and Death Investigation: Through the Eyes of the Forensic Nurse Practitioner. Dade County, FL, Metropolitan Dade County Medical Examiner Office, 1996.
6. Lynch VA: Keys to the Crime: Evidence Collection in Trauma. Lewisville, TX, Barbara Clark Mims Associates, 1991.
7. McCracken LM: Living forensics: A natural evolution in emergency care. Accid Emerg Nurs 7(4):211–216, 1999.
8. Prentky RA, Burgess AW: Forensic Management of Sexual Offenders. New York, Kluwer Academic Publishers, 2000.
9. Spitz WU, et al: Medico-legal Investigation of Death: Guidelines for the Application of Pathology to Crime Investigation, 3rd ed. Springfield, IL, Charles C Thomas, 1993.
10. Standing Bear ZG: Forensic nursing and death investigation: Will the vision be co-opted? J Psychol Nurs Mental Health Serv 33(9):59–64, 1995.
11. Swan KG, Swan RC: Gunshot Wounds: Pathophysiology and Management, 2nd ed. Chicago, Year-Book, 1989.
12. Winfrey ME, Smith AR: Confronting forensic issues. Crit Care Nurs Q 22(1):1–7, 1999.
13. Winfrey ME, Smith AR: The suspiciousness factor: Critical care nursing and forensics. Crit Care Nurs Q 22(1):1–7, 1999.

6. INJURY PREVENTION

Bobette G. Henslee, RN, BSN, CCRN

1. Why should a trauma nurse be concerned with preventing injuries outside the hospital?

Perhaps you, as the trauma nurse, are considered the "authority" on injury prevention in your family, neighborhood, church, parent-teacher association, club, or social circle. Do you feel prepared to answer all of the questions that you field? Information is available in many, widespread locations. This chapter attempts to compile relevant information that you can use to educate yourself and others.

SAFETY ON WHEELS

2. Why should children have to wear a bicycle helmet?

Research has shown that, when worn correctly, bicycle helmets reduce the risk of serious head injury by approximately 85% and the risk of brain injury by approximately 88%. Even "minor" head injuries have been shown to produce problems with memory and learning over the long term. Head injury is the primary or contributing cause in 70–80% of all bicycle-related deaths. Many states in the U.S. and many countries worldwide now have mandatory bicycle helmet laws for children. Check local statutes and ordinances to be sure.

3. Can a bicycle helmet be used safely for in-line skating?

Although one helmet will work for both bicycling and in-line skating, serious skaters should consider a helmet that offers better protection for the back of the head, the most likely area of the head to hit the ground during skating. In-line skating helmets have more shock-absorbing Styrofoam that extends lower down the back.

4. Explain the significance of the sticker statement, "complies with CPSC standard," which is found on the inside of bike helmets.

As of February 1999, all bicycle helmets sold in the United States have to meet new federal safety standards set by the Consumer Product Safety Commission (CPSC). This statement attests that the helmet meets the CPSC standard.

5. In addition to adjusting the straps, how can I make the bicycle helmet fit even better?

The helmet should fit snugly and can be customized by using thinner or thicker removable foam pads inside. Extra pads that come with the helmet should be saved because the thick pads that a child can use now may need to be exchanged for thinner pads at a later time as the child grows.

6. How can I check the fit of the helmet?

With the strap buckled, gently try to move the helmet around on the head. The helmet should not move more than $\frac{1}{2}$ inch in any direction, especially backward; excessive movement exposes the forehead to injury in a crash.

7. Where do the two plastic pieces on the side straps of the helmet fit?

The plastic pieces on the two side straps (at the V of the straps) should fit just under the ears.

8. How far back on the head should the helmet sit?

A bicycle helmet should sit on the top of the head, low on the forehead, and just above the eyebrows without sliding backward.

9. My helmet seems to choke me. How much space can safely be allowed between the strap and the chin?

The buckle should be just under the chin, with about one finger's width of space between the strap and the chin. The strap should be comfortably snug but still allow the mouth to be opened.

10. Can an older helmet that has a fabric covering on the outside still be used?

The smooth plastic covering of current helmets helps hold the Styrofoam together as it crushes in a crash and helps the helmet to slide easily along the pavement. A cloth covering can snag on the pavement in a slide. An older helmet (manufactured before the CPSC standards were mandated) with a plastic covering may still be used if it has not been in a crash as long as it has a sticker on the inside demonstrating compliance with voluntary Snell standards or voluntary standards from the American Society for Testing and Materials or American National Standards Institute (ANSI).

11. Where can helmets for a larger-than-average head be found?

Several manufacturers have extra large helmets. One model fits a head circumference of up to 26 inches (66 cm). Bicycle stores may be able to order a larger helmet.

12. When should a helmet be replaced?

According to the Bicycle Helmet Safety Institute, a helmet must be replaced after any crash in which the rider's head is struck. The Styrofoam part is made for "one-crash" use. After crushing it is no longer as protective as it was, even if it still looks intact. Plastic shells can hide the foam damage. If in doubt, contact the manufacturer for an inspection. If the helmet is more than 10 years old or has a cloth cover, it should be replaced. Many manufacturers recommend replacement after 5 years. Deterioration depends on usage, care, and abuse.

13. How can loosening of the strap be prevented?

Some straps loosen after just one ride. Look for a helmet with wider rather than thinner straps. Rubber O-rings can be added to the straps to slide up against the buckle and secure the strap when it is adjusted to fit correctly. Once you have the perfect fit, the ends of the straps can be sewn in place.

14. How does the light-weight Styrofoam in a helmet provide protection?

When you crash and hit a hard surface, the Styrofoam part of the helmet crushes, absorbing some of the crash energy and increasing the time it takes for the rider's head to stop by about six hundredths of a second. Thus the peak impact to the brain is reduced. Thicker Styrofoam is better, giving your head more of a cushion.

15. What advice must be given to the bicyclist wearing an unbuckled helmet?

Always buckle the helmet before riding so that it will not fall off or move out of position.

16. What is a good rule of thumb for bicycling in the street?

Bicyclists generally are safest when they act and are treated as drivers of motor vehicles. In some areas, bicycles are considered vehicles by law when operated in the street and must follow all traffic rules applying to motor vehicles. Check local statutes and ordinances to be sure.

17. How can I tell if a bicycle is too big for the driver?

As the driver of a bike, one should be able to straddle the bike comfortably in the standing position, with both feet flat on the ground. When the driver is sitting on the seat, the tips of the toes should be able to touch the ground.

18. In the United States, when can a bicyclist legally be in any area of the roadway other than the right side?

In most areas (when no bike lane is available), bicyclists may legally ride anywhere in the roadway under the following conditions:

- If they are not impeding traffic
- To avoid hazards
- To pass vehicles or other bicycles
- To prepare for a left turn

Check local statutes and ordinances to be sure.

19. Can a bicyclist use the left-turn lane?

In most areas, a bicyclist may legally use a left-turn lane just like the driver of a motor vehicle. Check local statutes and ordinances to be sure. Use of the right-turn lane is appropriate in countries such as Great Britain, where motor vehicles drive on the left side of the road.

20. What suggestions may improve safety of the bicyclist who travels at night?

Many more motor vehicle–bicycle collisions occur at night than in the daylight hours. If you ride during darkness, wear bright colors, reflective clothing and/or stickers, and use a front light and reflectors on your bike. You definitely want to be noticed. Be sure to obey all laws, and be extra careful!

21. Of what potential dangers should a bicyclist be aware when approaching an intersection?

Many crashes occur when cars turn into the path of a bicycle. Do not pass cars on the right at intersections, and watch for cars turning right (and drivers looking to the left for oncoming traffic) when crossing the intersection. In countries such as Great Britain caution is advised to watch for cars turning left.

22. How should the driver of a motor vehicle pass a bicyclist?

A motorist should pass bicycles safely by leaving at least 3 feet of space between the car and the bicycle. The motorist should slow down and use the next lane if necessary (and avoid honking the horn!). Be extra careful on windy days, because the steering of a bicycle is easily affected by wind.

23. What is the number-one injury associated with skateboarding?

According to the National Safety Council, wrist injury (usually a fracture or sprain).

24. What safety equipment can help reduce injuries related to skateboarding?

Helmets, slip-resistant and closed-toe shoes, padded shorts and jackets, specialized padding for hips, knees, and elbows, wrist braces, and skateboarding gloves can help absorb the impact from a fall and reduce injury.

25. What can be done to reduce serious injury due to falls from skates and skateboards?

Learning how to fall and practicing fall techniques on soft surfaces may help reduce injuries.

26. What are the steps to learning how to fall?

The goal of learning to fall is landing on the fleshy parts of the body. When losing your balance, try to crouch as low to the ground as possible to shorten the distance of the fall. Rather than trying to break the fall with your hands or arms, try to roll with your arms close to the body. Also try to relax rather than stiffen the body, which is often the initial response.

27. What kind of difference does wearing a helmet make for the motorcyclist?

In 1999, helmets were approximately 29% effective in preventing motorcycle deaths and about 67% effective in preventing brain injuries, according to the U.S. National Highway Traffic Safety Association (NHTSA).

28. How much more likely is an unhelmeted motorcycle rider to suffer a fatal head injury than a helmeted rider?

Compared with a helmeted rider, an unhelmeted rider is approximately 40% more likely to suffer a fatal head injury.

29. How does the death rate of motorcyclists compare with the death rate of people in automobiles?

According to NHTSA's Traffic Safety Facts 1999, the number of motorcycle crash-related deaths per mile traveled is about 16 times the number of motor vehicle crash-related deaths.

30. What are the more common areas of injury for motorcyclists?

Face, chest, lower leg, skull, and cervical spine.

31. Do the "shorty" helmets, which look more like a baseball cap than a motorcycle helmet, provide adequate protection for a motorcyclist's head?

Small helmets are labeled and sold exclusively as novelty items. Similar-looking helmets comply with the U.S. Department of Transportation (DOT) safety standard for use with a motorized cycle. Check the inside or back of the helmet for a DOT safety label. A full facial-shield protective motorcycle helmet that complies with the DOT standard offers more protection for the face and head than the abbreviated helmets.

MOTOR VEHICLE SAFETY

32. Why do most safety professionals take pains to avoid using the word *accident*?

Most crashes are not accidents. The word *accident* promotes the concept of random events over which we have no control. The fact is that many "accidents" are not only preventable but also predictable. The word *accident* implies that the resulting injuries are an unavoidable part of our lives. The words *crash, collision, incident*, and *injury* should be promoted as more appropriate substitutes.

33. What percentage of traffic crashes or incidents involve fire or submersion?

Less than 1%.

34. Does a safety restraint make it more likely that an occupant will be trapped in a submerged vehicle?

The restrained occupant of a submerged vehicle is more likely to remain conscious and to be able to escape the vehicle.

35. Will a lap and shoulder restraint always protect a driver from striking the steering wheel?

No. If the driver sits too close to the steering wheel, the head may strike the wheel even if the upper body is held off the steering wheel by the restraint. A general rule of thumb is to sit at least 10 inches from the steering wheel, with or without a driver's side air bag.

36. When a parent's restraint belt is buckled, how often are children traveling in the same vehicle also buckled?

According to NHTSA, in 98% of cases.

37. Apart from staying off the road entirely, what is the best protection against an impaired driver?
Wearing a safety belt.

38. How often are children unbuckled when the parent is unbuckled?
According to NHTSA, in about 46% of cases.

39. What is the best way to increase child restraint use?
By increasing adult restraint use. Children model adult behavior. Adults should set a good example for children riding with them in motor vehicles.

40. What is the best way to increase adult restraint use?
The passage of primary belt use laws in state after state has proved to increase safety belt usage and to reduce injuries and deaths.

41. What can be done to keep a shoulder belt from rubbing across the neck of a small child (aged 4–8 years)?
Using a booster seat to raise the child often keeps the shoulder belt from rubbing across the neck. Belt positioning boosters have a strap or guide to direct the belt away from the neck. Built-in shoulder belt height adjusters in some vehicles also may improve the fit. If the belt still rubs the neck, put a soft cloth around the belt to increase comfort and to reduce the risk that the child will slip the belt under his or her arm or behind the body when no one is watching.

42. How helpful are add-on seat belt adjusters?
Add-on shoulder belt adjusters are not controlled or tested to federal standards. In some cases, they make seat belts less effective by allowing the lap belt to ride up higher on the abdomen. An add-on shoulder belt adjuster should not be used instead of a car seat or booster seat. Make sure that the child never puts the shoulder belt under the arm or behind the back; both of these positions have the potential for causing serious injury.

43. How do I know that a lap belt fits correctly?
The lap belt should fit low and tight across the top of the thighs, not up on the abdomen. If the child is sitting on bench seats or is too short to sit straight with the knees bending naturally over the edge of the seat, the lap belt will probably ride up over the abdomen, increasing risk of injury. A poor fitting lap belt can result in serious abdominal and spinal injuries.

44. How do I know that a shoulder belt fits correctly?
The shoulder belt should be worn across the middle of the shoulder and chest. If the belt cuts across the throat and cannot be adjusted, try tilting the seat back slightly for an adult. If the belt cuts across the throat of a child, it is generally a sign of a poor fit. A booster seat to raise the child will improve the fit into an adult lap/shoulder belt.

45. The back seat is said to be the safest location in a vehicle. Which position in the back seat is the safest?
The center of the rear seats is the safest because it blocks intrusion from either side. More and more vehicle manufacturers are installing lap/shoulder belts in the middle seating position, which make it even safer. A child in a child restraint can be restrained in the middle rear seat with only a lap belt, if no other restraint is available in that position. A belt-positioning booster seat, which is not technically considered a child restraint but rather a child booster, needs the use of both lap and shoulder belts. Shield or tray boosters can be used in a lap belt-only position but do not provide the best upper body protection. However, a shield or tray booster is better protection than a poorly fitting lap belt.

46. Can the lap belt of the center-rear seat in an older car be retrofitted to add a shoulder belt?

The anchorage for the center-rear shoulder belt must be designed into the vehicle. There is no way to add a shoulder belt in the center back seat of most current models.

47. Can shoulder belts and tether anchors be retrofitted into rear-seating positions of pre-1990 cars?

Some vehicle manufacturers offer model-specific retrofit kits to add tether anchors and shoulder belts. Check with the vehicle dealer. Dealership personnel may be unaware of these kits and may have to call the manufacturer. The manufacturer indemnifies dealers for the installations with kits made specifically for the vehicles that they carry. If the dealer personnel install the kits according to directions, they are not liable for damages. For a free copy of a NHTSA pamphlet (DOT HS 807811, 11/92) that lists most available retrofit kits, contact Safety-Belt Safe U.S.A. at P.O. Box 553, Altadena, CA 91003, at (800) 745-7233, or at www.carseat.org. Ask for pamphlet 428. Chrysler kits are listed at www.childsafety.org.

48. How much force are safety belts built to withstand?

Safety restraints are built to withstand about 6000 pounds of force acting on them in a crash.

49. What is so significant about crash forces?

Because many different factors affect the amount of force involved in a crash (e.g., vehicle type, object struck, precrash maneuvering), accurate calculations can be quite complex. In the *Standardized Child Passenger Safety Training Manual*, NHTSA describes a conservative rule of thumb approximation: The force to restrain is approximately equal to the child's weight times vehicle speed before the crash. For example, in a motor vehicle moving at 30 mph (48 kPH), at least 600 pounds of force may be required to restrain a 20-pound infant from moving. During the crash an infant held in an adult's arms will become so heavy that it cannot possibly be restrained. Each person, adult or child, riding in a vehicle requires his or her own restraint. No sharing should be allowed, especially with safety belts, tether anchors, and straps.

50. Do safety belts have to be replaced after use in a crash?

Seat belts, child restraints, and air bags are considered "'one-crash use" products. After use in a crash they must be replaced. Vehicle manufacturers recommend replacement of seat belts except in cases of minor crashes. Because of the many factors involved in a crash, it is hard to determine whether a specific collision speed is necessary to cause damage. See a qualified auto technician to determine whether the belts and any involved tether anchors have been damaged in the crash.

51. In 2002, how many people in the U.S. can expect to be involved in motor vehicle crashes?

Approximately one in eight people.

52. At what approximate speed and distance from home do most traffic fatalities occur in the U.S.?

More than 80% of all U.S. traffic crashes occur at speeds less than 40 mph (64 kPH), and 3 of 4 crashes causing deaths occur within 25 miles of home.

53. What is the leading cause of death for children (5–14 years old) of all races in the U.S.?

Motor vehicle crashes.

54. At night, what happens when a car travels so fast that it overdrives the headlights and cannot stop inside the illuminated area?

A blind crash area is created in front of the vehicle.

55. Why is twilight one of the most challenging times to drive?

The driver's eyes are attempting to adapt to the growing darkness.

56. What visual clues can alert you to the possibility of an impaired driver?

Drivers who are impaired often straddle the center line, weave between the lines, make wide turns, stop abruptly, have difficulty in maintaining a consistent speed, or respond slowly to traffic signals.

57. What evasive actions can be taken to avoid an impaired driver on the roadway?

If you notice some of the behaviors of an impaired driver, leave the roadway at the nearest exit or turn at the nearest corner. Try to get the vehicle's description or license plate, and report it to law enforcement as soon as possible.

58. What evasive actions can be taken to avoid an oncoming vehicle that crosses into your lane?

If it appears that an oncoming car is crossing into your lane, pull over to the roadside, sound the horn, and flash your lights.

59. What are some of the warning signs of driver fatigue?

Staring straight ahead in a trance-like state at a monotonous roadway ("highway hypnosis"), burning eyes, back tension, shallow breathing, and inattentiveness are some of the warning signs of driver fatigue. Other signs include some of the same behaviors exhibited by impaired drivers, such as any kind of erratic driving, difficulty in maintaining a consistent speed, responding slowly to traffic signals, drifting, tailgating, and failure to obey traffic signs.

60. Apart from pulling off the road to rest, what can the tired driver do to combat fatigue?

- Adjust the ambiance inside the vehicle so that it helps keep you awake (e.g, open the windows, use minimal air conditioning in summer and minimal heat in winter).
- Turn up the radio volume, and switch stations frequently.
- Talk to yourself, or sing.
- Take note of other vehicles around you; keep your eyes moving.
- Keep your body involved in the driving by avoiding cruise control and varying speed.
- Stretch your legs, take breaks at least every 2 hours, and eat light snacks, avoiding alcohol.

61. What principles about young children and traffic should drivers keep in mind?

Children under the age of 8 years often think that if they can see the driver of a vehicle, the driver can also see them. Young children do not always recognize danger, understand cause and effect, or respond appropriately. They may have difficulty in judging how fast traffic is moving and often think that vehicles can stop immediately. Young children also have difficulty in locating sounds and are highly distractible.

62. As a nurse caring for pediatric patients, how can I help young children understand about traffic hazards?

Generally speaking, children under age 8 years should cross streets only with an adult and should walk through parking lots while holding an adult's hand. Talk to children about street safety, and show them how to stop at the curb or edge of the street, looking to the left, to the right, and then to the left again before crossing the street. (In countries such as Great Britain, the child should look right, left, and right again.) Children model adult behavior; set a good example for your child. Children who are too young to know left from right can be taught to look "this way, that way, and this way again."

63. Is there a nationally recognized resource for multicultural traffic safety information?

NHTSA offers multicultural information at www.nhtsa.dot.gov.

AIR BAG SAFETY

64. How do you know if a vehicle has frontal, side impact, or head restraint air bags?

Look for air bag warning labels on the steering wheel hub, windshield, instrument panel, air bag cover, front or back of the sun visor, dashboard, vehicle door frame, door panels, seat belt, side or back of the vehicle seat, and in the vehicle owner's manual.

65. What do all of those letters on the air bag covers mean?
- SRS = supplemental restraint system
- SIR = supplemental inflatable restraint
- SIPS = side-impact protection system
- SIAB = side-impact air bag
- IC = inflatable curtain

All of these letters indicate the presence of air bags.

66. Where are side-impact air bags located in vehicles?

Side-impact air bags may be found in both front and rear seating positions and may be mounted in the door, in the seat or on the side of the seat, in the column between doors, or over the window. Consult the owner's manual, and look for warning labels.

67. How and why do air bags inflate so forcefully?

When the air bag is triggered, sodium azide tablets are ignited and generate a large amount of nitrogen gas, leading to air-bag inflation in approximately 30–40 milliseconds. Air bags need to inflate rapidly so that the occupant contacts a fully inflated bag (buffering cushion) rather than the interior of the vehicle. As the air bag quickly deflates, crash force energy is absorbed and spread over a larger surface area, reducing the risk of injuries.

68. Are more than just frontal driver and passenger air bags available?

Some vehicle manufacturers offer frontal knee air bags and frontal foot air bags.

69. What makes the air bag deploy?

Crash sensors located on the front of the vehicle and in the passenger compartment measure deceleration of the vehicle. When sensors reach a deceleration threshold, an electronic signal is sent to the inflator and triggers deployment of the air bag.

70. What types and angles of motor vehicle crashes cause a deployment of frontal air bags?

Frontal air bags are designed to deploy in moderate-to-severe frontal crashes (from the center of the vehicle at 0° to about a 30° angle from the center).

71. What degree of crash force triggers frontal air bag deployment?

Frontal air bag deployment is triggered when the crash forces are about equivalent to striking a brick wall head-on at 10–12 mph (16–19 kPH) or, in a similar-sized vehicle, at approximately 20–30 mph (32–48 kPH). Thresholds of 10–12 mph (16–19 kPH) may be used for unrestrained occupants, but thresholds may be higher (about 16 mph [26 kPH]) for people with safety restraints because they may be less likely to be injured in crashes at slower speeds.

72. What about frontal air bag deployment in other types of crashes?

Frontal air bags are not designed to deploy in side-impact, rear-impact, or roll-over crashes.

73. How long does an air bag remain inflated?
Measured holes in the air bag allow the gases to escape quickly (over milliseconds) and to begin the deflation process.

74. Can an air bag deploy after the engine is turned off?
There have been instances when an air bag deployed several minutes to several hours after the vehicle battery had been disconnected.

75. Can an air bag be used again after it has been deployed in a crash?
Like seat belts and child restraint systems, an air bag is used once in a crash and then must be replaced.

76. Who regulates air bags?
NHTSA regulates frontal air bags. At present it does not regulate side-impact air bags.

77. Do any vehicles come equipped with an on/off switch for the passenger air bag?
Some two-seater cars and most regular cab and extended-cab pickup trucks come equipped with an on/off switch for the passenger air bag. Drivers can transport an infant in a rear-facing child seat when the switch is turned off. However, the switch must be turned on again to protect adult passengers. Therefore, these types of vehicles should not be considered for routine family transportation.

78. What is the procedure for obtaining permission to have an air bag on/off switch installed?
People wishing to have an air bag on/off switch must read an informational brochure, "Air Bags & On-Off Switches: Information for an Informed Decision." A separate request form should be completed, then sent to NHTSA.

79. How can I obtain the paperwork for the air bag on/off switch?
The brochure and separate request form are available from the Auto Safety Hotline (1-888-DASH-2-DOT) or at www.nhtsa.dot.gov.

80. Who can install the air bag on/off switch?
Automobile dealers may install on/off air bag switches. Many dealers have refused to install them even if the NHTSA grants authorization.

81. How do side air bags affect child safety?
At present, correctly restrained child passengers, properly positioned in the vehicle and the seat, do not seem to be at risk of injury from side air bags. However, some manufacturers think that a child who is unrestrained or out of position can be injured. They have produced "smart" side air bags that sense when an occupant is too close. NHTSA recommends that children should not be placed next to the side air bag unless the vehicle manufacturer specifically states that it is safe to do so or the air bag has been disconnected. Some child restraint manufacturers advise against placing the car seat next to a side air bag. Check the vehicle and child restraint owner's manuals.

82. If a child is seated on a booster next to a side-impact air bag, is he or she at risk for injury if the side air bag deploys?
Yes. "Properly restrained" means sitting upright, not leaning or slouching against the door. Note the child's behavior in the seat. Is the child able to sit without slouching and leaning? Check the vehicle and booster seat owner's manuals for any warnings against placing the seat next to a side air bag.

83. At approximately what speed does the driver's air bag deploy?
At speeds of up to approximately 140 mph (224 kPH).

84. At approximately what speed does the passenger air bag deploy?

At speeds up to approximately 200 mph (320 kPH). The passenger air bag is about twice the size and comes out twice as far as the driver's air bag. The higher deployment speed is necessary to inflate the bag fully in milliseconds.

85. How far away from a steering wheel should a driver sit, with or without an air bag?

A driver should allow at least 10 inches of space between the center of the steering wheel and the center of the breastbone. This minimal space should allow the air bag to inflate fully; it also allows enough room to keep the head from striking the steering wheel even as the upper body is restrained with a shoulder belt.

86. What can drivers of short stature do to put enough distance between themselves and the steering wheel?

A shorter driver may try tilting the seat back and adjusting the steering wheel upward after pulling the seat as far back as possible. Drivers who cannot put enough distance between themselves and the steering wheel may consider using pedal extenders or requesting installation of an air bag on/off switch.

87. How far from the air bag should the front-seat passenger sit?

At least 24 inches of space should be maintained between the dashboard and the passenger in the front seat. Because the passenger air bag is twice the size of the driver air bag, the passenger seat should be pulled all the way back for safety.

88. Can I have my air bags turned off?

As of January 1998, consumers can choose to have an air bag on/off switch installed if they or a user of their vehicle belongs to an at-risk group.

89. Define at-risk groups.

- People who must transport infants in rear-facing infant seats or children aged 12 and under in the front passenger seat
- Drivers who cannot maintain 10 inches of space between the center of the steering wheel and the center of their sternum
- People whose doctors confirm that, because of their medical condition, the air bag poses a special risk that outweighs the risk of hitting the head, neck, or chest in a crash if the air bag is turned off

90. Are small adults and children at greater risk of air bag injury because of their size?

Air bag injuries occur most often when vehicle occupants are positioned improperly in relation to the inflating air bag, not because of size or age. Most air bag-related deaths involve people who were not wearing safety belts, were improperly belted, or were positioned improperly in the vehicle seat.

91. Who at the national level is collecting side air-bag crash information?

Emergency rescue personnel are encouraged to notify NHTSA of a side air-bag crash, Call the Special Crash Investigation Hotline at (202) 493-0400; fax to (202) 366-5374; or e-mail to air bag.crash@nhtsa.dot.gov.

CHILD PASSENGER SAFETY

92. What is a basic principle of child passenger safety?

The field of child passenger safety is a complex and constantly changing field. In fact, although the information presented here is current as this book goes to press, some of the more technical information may become outdated quickly. Keeping up to date is key. Keeping current about new products, research, and best practices is challenging, but many resources are available. An excellent resource is *Safe Ride News*, a subscriber-funded, bimonthly publication available in print and electronic form. *Safe Ride News* articles are more comprehensive and cover more than just technical issues. There is also a child passenger safety (CPS) listserve on which related issues are discussed at CPSPList@yahoogroups.com.

93. To reduce potential legal liability, what is the best response to a question or situation related to child restraint safety with which you are unfamiliar?

When you do not know the answer or the issue is unclear, be willing to say, "I don't know, but I will try to find out" or "I can't tell you a safe way to do that." It is important to recognize your limits and admit that you do not know or are unsure of an answer. Be sure to contact the network of CPS technicians in your area to determine an answer for the parents.

94. What general recommendation can a trauma nurse make to all parents of children riding in child restraints?

Advise parents to read both the car seat's and the vehicle's owner's manuals. If they still have questions, encourage them to have the child safety seats inspected by a certified child safety seat technician. To find a nearby inspection location or a certified child passenger safety technician, call 866-SEAT CHECK or visit www.seatcheck.org.

95. To what degree does proper use of a child restraint reduce fatality rates?

Research estimates that infant fatalities can be reduced by 71% and toddler fatalities by 54% when child restraints are used properly. Further estimates indicate that about 69% of child crash-related hospitalizations could be avoided with proper child restraint usage. These figures are significant considering that approximately 80% of child restraints are not properly installed.

96. What two booklets should be consulted before installing a child restraint into a vehicle?

The child restraint owner's manual and the vehicle owner's manual should be read thoroughly.

97. Why should a rear-facing infant restraint not be used in the front seat if a passenger air bag is installed?

The inflating air bag strikes the seat with such force that the infant can be critically injured or killed.

98. What is the safest direction to face when riding in a vehicle?

According to the NHTSA, facing backward—unless, of course, you are driving!

99. Why must an infant child restraint face the rear of the vehicle?

The back of the rear-facing infant seat supports the head, neck, and back in a crash. If an infant is facing forward in a crash, the heavy head may be pulled away from the body with more force than the immature bones and ligaments of the neck can safely withstand. Serious or fatal injury can result. In addition, the side wings of the seat help to keep the rear-facing infant's head contained within the confines of the shell. This design helps to prevent head injury in side-impact crashes.

100. Why must an infant's seat be reclined when placed in a moving vehicle?

To reduce the risk of neck injury in the event of a crash, to maintain an open airway, and to make the infant more comfortable. The recline angle of the seat should not be more than 45° from vertical for small infants. As the infant grows and control of the neck muscles develops, the seat can be adjusted to a more semiupright position, enhancing the child's comfort while maintaining safety.

101. Why are infants at risk for positional apnea in a child restraint?

An infant's head is too heavy for neck muscles that are not strong enough to keep the head upright at all times. The head can flop forward and occlude the airway, causing positional apnea. Therefore, a recline angle of no more than 45° from vertical is recommended for young infants.

102. What is the purpose of the recline indicator on the side of the infant seat?

The recline indicator helps to maintain the angle of recline at no more than 45° from vertical. A tightly rolled small towel or blanket or a section (cut to fit) of a foam swimming pool "noodle" can help to fill the gap where the vehicle seat back and bottom meet the infant restraint base. This strategy helps to maintain the proper angle of infant restraint recline.

103. Why recline an infant's seat no more than 45° from vertical? Why not place the infant in a flat lying position?

A seat back that is reclined too far in the rear-facing position can cause the infant to move up the back of the seat in a crash. Thus, too much force is loaded onto the infant's shoulders, or the infant could slide out of the harness straps headfirst in a crash.

104. Is a more upright position better for crash protection?

Yes, but this principle must be balanced by the need to maintain an open airway and the infant's comfort. As infants develop and their neck muscles become stronger, they can be positioned at a more upright angle.

105. What signs may indicate that the infant needs a greater degree of recline?

If the head of a sleeping or young infant appears to fall away from the shell of the seat, the airway may become occluded and greater G force may be exerted on the head in a crash; thus, more recline (but no more than 45° from vertical) is indicated.

106. Why do some parents turn the child seat to face forward before the child reaches its first birthday or exceeds the weight limit for riding in a rear-facing position?

By the time infants reach 6–8 months of age, they can usually sit up alone and may struggle to sit more upright in the child restraint. Parents often conclude that the child's seat can be turned to a forward-facing position. Outdated child restraint instructions and pamphlets may indicate that children can ride in a forward-facing position when they can sit upright. It is permissible to keep a child in the rear-facing position until the maximal weight limit is reached. However, most parents are eager to turn the child to a forward-facing position so that they can keep an eye on the child more easily. Remind parents who are nervous about having the child out of sight that riding in the back seat in a rear-facing position is safest not only for the child but also for the driver, who is less distracted from the road. If the child needs attention, the only safe choice is to pull off the road and attend to the child.

107. Which child restraint system is best?

All child restraints that are certified to meet federal safety standards must perform at a certain level. According to NHTSA, the best seat is the one that fits the child and the vehicle and will be used correctly for every ride.

108. Are convertible child restraints with a T-shield or tray safe to use with a small infant?

The American Academy of Pediatrics advises that a small infant should not be placed in a child restraint with a shield, abdominal pad, or armrest that can contact the face and neck during a crash. Handles of infant carriers should be positioned away from the child during transport in a vehicle for the same reason. Some parents think that these structures help to protect them in a crash, but they can actually cause injury.

109. Can the the padding and cover of a child restraint be removed for cleaning?

Some coverings may be removed and laundered. However, the covering may shrink and no longer fit the restraint. Check the manufacturer's instructions. Cleaning the cover while it is attached to the child restraint is the best way to avoid shrinkage.

110. How should an infant be positioned in a car seat?

An infant should be placed with the buttocks and back flat against the back of the seat. Blanket rolls may be placed on both sides of the infant to provide side support for the head and neck. Shoulder straps must be in the lowest slots until the infant's shoulders are above the slots; the harness must be snug (no more than one finger should fit between the strap and the infant's shoulder); and the retainer clip is positioned at the midpoint of the chest or armpit level. Extra padding should not be placed *under* a child in a car seat because it can compress in a crash, allowing more room between the child and the restraint straps. The child may come out of the seat headfirst. Any added padding should be no thicker than a placemat ($< \frac{1}{2}$ inch).

111. What visual clues indicate that a child has outgrown a forward-facing restraint?

When a child's shoulders extend above the top harness slots or the mid-point of the back of the head extends above the top of the shell.

112. Why are child restraints for use up to 40 pounds and with a full harness preferable to shield boosters?

Shield boosters were designed for use in seated positions with lap belts only. However, they provide limited upper body protection. Even though the shield booster and lap belt restrain the child at the hips, the child's upper body moves forward and can fold around the shield. A harness restrains the upper body better and is recommended for children under 40 pounds.

113. Is the performance of a rear-facing child restraint negatively affected if it touches the back of the seat in front of it?

In most cases, rear-facing seats can be installed so that they rest against the back of the vehicle seat ahead, unless manufacturer's instructions advise against this practice. If the gap is small or the child is on the heavy side, it is better for the seat to touch any forward structure before a crash than to hit it during the crash. Resting against a forward seat back is only one way to achieve these benefits. Another option is a seat with a tether specifically designed to be routed rearward to limit forward rotation of the seat. Check the seat manufacturer's instructions and vehicle owner's manual for tether anchorage information.

114. What advice can be given to parents struggling to keep their children restrained?

Unfortunately, there is no "escape-proof" child restraint. Because children often model their behavior after their parents, parents can create the buckle-up habit by buckling up themselves. Other parents have successfully introduced the "car seat interlock" routine. The idea is that an imaginary ignition interlock makes the car stop if anyone is not buckled. If the child gets out of the seat, the car stops and does not restart until the child is restrained again. Proper behavior should be positively reinforced. Boredom is often part of the restlessness problem in the child who cannot see out of the vehicle. Special "car toys" that are soft and small (e.g., picture books, favorite tapes) and frequent stops on long trips help to keep children happy in their seats.

115. Is it advisable to tether an older child restraint not originally designed for tethering?

A child restraint should never be tethered without the manufacturer's authorization. The place where the tether is attached may break if it was not designed to withstand crash forces.

116. Can a high-back booster seat be tethered to increase stability?

Check the child restraint owner's manual. Some high-back boosters can be tethered. Used with the internal harness (for children under 40 pounds in the U.S., 48 pounds in Canada), a tether reduces head excursion (movement of the head) in a crash. When used as a booster, the lap and shoulder belts restrain the child, but the tether helps to keep the seat stable.

117. Why tether a child restraint?

Tether straps, along with safety belts, keep child restraints in place and reduce the chance of head injury or other serious injury to the child. Used with forward-facing restraints, a tether reduces both forward and side-to-side movement. However, any child restraint that complies with the federal standards (FMVSS 213) must meet a minimal standard without use of the tether. Adding a tether improves performance.

118. In what situations does using the tether that came with the child restraint help to install the seat correctly?

- The safety belt will not stay tight when used according to installation instructions.
- Safety belts are mounted forward of the seat "bight" (where the back and seat cushions meet), allowing more than 1 inch of movement from side to side when the child restraint is pulled at the base.
- Contoured bucket seats prevent a tight installation.
- Rear seats have limited space for forward motion in a crash, as in many subcompact cars and pick-up trucks with rear seats.
- Child restraint is installed in a lap belt-seating position. Installation with a lap/shoulder belt improves performance for some child restraints, such as those with a shoulder belt lock-off.

119. When are children generally large enough to fit properly into an adult safety belt?

As a general guideline, NHTSA recommends that a booster seat be used until lap and shoulder belts fit correctly, often at about age 8.

120. Is my child big enough to use a safety belt?

Take the Safety-Belt Safe U.S.A. five-step test:
1. Does the child sit all the way back against the vehicle seat?
2. Do the child's knees bend comfortably at the edge of the vehicle seat?
3. Is the lap belt on the tops of the thighs?
4. Is the shoulder belt centered on the shoulder and chest?
5. Can the child stay seated in this position for the whole trip?

If you answered "no" to any of these questions, your child needs a booster seat to ride safely in the car. Riding in a booster is more comfortable for the child, may reduce squirming in the seat, and allows the child to see out of the vehicle more easily.

121. What happens to the head of a restrained, forward-facing occupant in a crash?

Research has shown that when a car crashes into a wall at a speed of 25–30 mph (40–48 kPH), the vehicle comes to an abrupt stop at a deceleration rate of about 20–25 G. The force exerted on the forward-facing child or adult's head can approach 60–70 G. This force pulls the head away from the body, and even strong neck muscles cannot keep the head connected to the neck. Instead, the stiffness of the bones together with connecting ligaments keeps the adult's head attached to the body. Young children have immature bones that are soft, and their neck can separate when pulled with force. Although the bones and ligaments of the infant's neck can be stretched up to 2 inches, the spinal cord can stretch only about $\frac{1}{4}$ inch before rupturing.

122. Why should a child restraint be covered when left unattended in a vehicle?

The plastic and exposed metal parts of a child restraint can become hot enough to burn when left in direct sunlight.

123. What is the extra metal device, resembling a sideways H, that comes with the car seat?

This device is a regular locking clip and is used to prevent slow loosening of the safety belt holding the child restraint. The tougher, heavy-duty "belt-shortening clip" is provided by an automobile manufacturer and is used to shorten a lap belt that does not lock.

124. Where should a regular locking clip be placed?

A regular locking clip is placed onto the lap and shoulder belt (grasped together) on the buckle side of the child restraint about an inch from the latch plate. If a locking clip binds against the lip of the shell or frame of the child restraint and cannot be moved any closer to the latch plate, the clip should be moved from the latch plate only as far as necessary to allow it to rest just inside the frame or shell.

125. Why not put the locking clip on the door-side of the child restraint where it is easiest to reach?

Placing the locking clip on the door-side of the restraint adds slack to the belt and may allow the locking clip to pop off during a crash, thus increasing risk of injury to the child.

126. I can barely wedge my child's safety restraint into my extended-cab pick-up truck. Is it acceptable for some of the seat's base to extend over the edge of the seat?

At least 80% of the child restraint base must contact and be supported by the vehicle seat cushion. This requirement may preclude using child restraints on the seat in the extended-cab area of pick-up trucks and on the center rear seat in cars with contoured bucket seats.

127. Can I use a child restraint on the jump seat of my extended-cab pick-up truck?

Because of their side-facing orientation, jump seats are not intended for use with child restraints. Child restraints are tested only in the forward-facing position. Most vehicle and child restraint manufacturers advise against using side-facing jump seats for the installation of child restraints.

128. What is LATCH?

Lower anchors and tethers for children (LATCH) is a new way of securing child restraints into vehicles without using the vehicle's safety belts. The system involves both the vehicle and the child restraint. Two lower metal bars are factory-installed at the seat bight (where the back cushion meets the seat cushion). The upper anchor, which may be a bar, strap, or bracket, is located behind the vehicle seat and used for tether attachment. LATCH-compatible child restraints have two straps that attach to the lower anchors. Most forward-facing restraints have the tether strap. It is unnecessary for booster seats to have the LATCH straps, nor is use of tethers required. This system makes installation of child restraints much easier.

129. My child restraint slides on both leather and cloth seats, even though the seat is tightly secured by safety belts. What can I do to prevent the sliding?

A thin rubber mesh pad (e.g., shelf liner) can help to reduce sliding of the child restraint and protect the vehicle seat (leather or cloth) if it does not interfere with how tightly the safety belt secures the seat. A tether also may help if the owner's instructions of the restraint and the vehicle do not advise against its use.

130. Can child restraints be used on an airplane?

Safety-Belt Safe recommends that parents find the wording on the label and in the owner's booklet stating that the restraint is certified for use in an airplane in case a flight attendant asks to see it. It is wise to call ahead to check the airline's policy and to avoid assignment to a seat in an exit row. Child restraints must be placed in a window seat so that they do not block the escape path and may not be used in an exit row. It is also wise to measure the restraint at the widest point to determine if it is wider than 17 inches. If so, it probably will not fit into a coach seat. Passengers who purchase a ticket for the child have the right to use a child restraint, but the airline can refuse to allow the restraint if the passenger hoped to use it in the nearest empty seat without purchasing a ticket. Several airlines offer significant discounts for children under 2 years of age. Because airplanes do not have shoulder belts, belt-positioning booster seats cannot be used. Harnesses and vests are not permitted. The Federal Aviation Association can provide additional information at http://www.faa.gov.

131. Where can a trauma nurse get training to become a certified CPS technician?
For information about standardized 32-hour CPS technician certification, contact the National Child Passenger Safety Board at http://www.cpsboard.org.

132. When do child safety seats expire?
The Juvenile Products Manufacturer's Association (JPMA) recommends 6 years. Some manufacturers suggest a life span of 5–6 years, and some have begun to stamp an expiration date on recent models. By general agreement, a seat that is 10 years old is too old. Beyond these general recommendations, there is no clear "best practice" at present.

133. Does the expiration period on the seat refer to date of manufacture or date of initial use?
At present there is no clear recommendation.

134. I cannot get a tight fit for the child restraint unless I twist the stalk of the safety belt to shorten the length. Does twisting a safety belt reduce its tensile strength significantly?
One study reported by the Society of Automotive Engineers tested safety belts untreated or soaked in either apple juice or cola and then dried. It was found that strength was reduced about 5% after one twist of the belt and about 10% after two full twists. Even twisted belts remained with at least two times the strength required by U.S. and E.C.E. standards. When untwisted, the belts returned to their 6000-pound strength.

PEDESTRIAN SAFETY

135. What is the second largest category of motor vehicle-related deaths?
Pedestrians struck by motor vehicles.

136. Which pedestrian group suffers the most motor vehicle–related fatalities: children or the elderly?
Children under age 16 years are most likely to be struck by motor vehicles, but the elderly are more likely to die after being struck by a motor vehicle.

137. More than one-half of pedestrian deaths in the U.S. in 1999 occurred in rural areas. What explains the higher ratio of deaths to injuries in rural areas?
Higher-impact speeds on rural roads.

138. What areas of the body are typically injured when a pedestrian is struck by a motor vehicle?
Knee, tibia, fibula, femur, pelvis, and vertebral column.

139. The greatest number of pedestrian deaths results from what mechanism of injury?
Pedestrians sustain the most serious injuries when they are thrown onto a vehicle's hood or windshield or onto the top of the vehicle.

140. At what location of the road or sidewalk do the majority of pedestrian deaths occur in people aged 65 and older?
More than one-third of deaths in elderly pedestrians occur at intersections.

141. On which two days of the week do most motor vehicle-related pedestrian deaths occur?
Friday and Saturday.

142. At what time of day do most fatal pedestrian-motor vehicle collisions occur?
Between 6 and 9 PM.

143. What does it mean when the walk signal at a crossing begins to flash?
The flashing "walk" signal has the same meaning as a steady "don't walk" signal: pedestrians should not begin crossing the street; they should wait for the next light cycle. The flashing signal allows enough time to cross if the pedestrian has already stepped into the street when the light begins to flash—no need to break into a run! However, elderly or physically impaired persons may not have enough time to finish crossing safely.

144. What should a pedestrian do when walking along a road with no sidewalks?
Pedestrians should walk facing traffic so that they can see oncoming cars. They should check for cars by looking both ways while walking and before crossing the street. When crossing the street, even if they have the right of way, pedestrians should yield to motor vehicles. It is always wise to make an extra effort to be seen. During the daytime, especially at dawn or dusk, pedestrians should attach reflective material to clothing, backpack, or purse and wear light or brightly colored clothing. At night, pedestrians should carry a flashlight; wear a reflective headband, armband, or vest; or attach a flashing light to clothing in front and back.

145. How much peripheral vision do children under age 10 have compared with adults?
Children under the age of 10 have about one-third the peripheral vision of adults.

146. Where should pedestrians cross the street if no crosswalks are provided?
At corners, where there are usually fewer obstructions to visibility. Children should be taught and reminded frequently never to cross the street between parked cars. A parked vehicle can greatly impair the child's ability to see and be seen by drivers.

147. How are toddlers (1 and 2 year olds) most often injured as pedestrians?
By a vehicle that is backing up. The driver may not see a child who is playing in a driveway or parking area.

148. How are preschoolers (3 and 4 year olds) most often struck by motor vehicles?
Preschoolers are hit most often when they dash across a street near home.

SENIOR SAFETY/FALL PREVENTION

149. What often leads to self-imposed restrictions on mobility in the elderly?
The constant fear of falling.

150. What tips can the trauma nurse give the elderly to prevent falls in the bathroom?
1. Install hand rails in the bath tub and toilet areas.
2. Bathroom rugs should have a nonskid backing.
3. Skid-resistant strips are also a good idea, especially in the tub.
4. Use locks on the bathroom door that can be opened from both sides to avoid being accidentally locked in the bathroom.

151. What advice can be given to elderly people who trip or frequently catch their feet on various objects?
These occurrences may mean that strength should be improved. Inactivity leads to lack of balance and weak muscles. Walking and dancing are ideal activities for improving balance and muscle strength. Choose stairs, not escalators, and walk whenever possible.

152. Research has shown that choosing the wrong chair can lead to hip fractures. What advice should be given to the elderly about choice of chair?

Choose chairs with arms and a seat at a 90° angle (or level with the knees). Chairs without arms that allow the buttocks to be lower than the knees can lead to hip fractures when the elderly rise from the chair improperly.

153. Can an elderly person fracture a hip while getting out of a car?

Yes. Care should be taken when getting out of cars because a motion similar to that described in question 152 puts abnormal pressure on the hip when the person stands up, potentially leading to a hip fracture.

154. What can elderly users of public transportation do to ensure their safety?

- Take your time getting on and off the vehicle; use the handrail.
- Have your fare ready so that you do not have to look for change as the vehicle starts to move.
- Brace yourself when the vehicle starts or slows down.
- Keep one hand free to grasp railings and brace yourself.
- Wear shoes that fit snugly.
- Avoid wearing long coats or skirts that may catch on your shoe as you ascend or descend steps.

155. What can be done about stairs to make them safer for the elderly?

- Install nonslip treads, good lighting, and a solid, easy-to-grasp handrail.
- Paint or tape the top and bottom steps so they are easily noticed.
- Advise the elderly not to rush when using stairs.
- Make sure that the walkway is clear.

156. After falls, what is the second leading cause of death for people age 65 and over?
Motor vehicle crashes.

157. What are the most common reasons that elderly people drown?

The most common reason is a fall into a canal, lake, or a pool, but poor health plays a part, as do alcohol consumption and suicide.

BURN SAFETY

158. What is the recommended temperature setting for a water heater to avoid scald burns?

Set the water heater temperature no higher than 120°F (49° Celsius) to prevent scald injuries. According to the National SAFE KIDS campaign, a child exposed to hot tap water at 140°F (60° C) for just 3 seconds will sustain a full-thickness burn, which requires hospitalization and skin grafts. In children, burns resulting from exposure to tap water cover a larger area of the body and are generally more severe.

159. Why are young children especially vulnerable to burn-related injury and death?

Young children often do not recognize danger, have a limited ability to react quickly and appropriately, and have less control over their surroundings. Because their skin is thinner than an adult's skin, burns occur at lower temperatures and are more severe.

160. In what area of the home do most scald burns, caused by water from the faucet, occur?

Most scald burns caused by tap water occur in the bathroom and are associated with more injuries and deaths to young children than burns caused by other hot liquids.

161. What should parents make sure that all members of the household are able to do in the event of a fire?
- Easily open all doors and windows
- Identify two escape routes from every room
- Meet outside the home at a designated place
- Practice the escape plan at least twice a year

162. Why is it important to crawl out of a smoke-filled area on your hands and knees rather than on your belly?
Poisons may settle in a thin layer on the floor.

163. Is one smoke detector in the home enough?
Every home should be equipped with smoke detectors on every floor and especially outside sleeping areas. Test batteries monthly and change batteries twice a year (with time changes).

164. How can occupants of a dwelling protect against an electrical fire?
If the lights in the home dim or flicker when extra electrical appliances are plugged in, the electrical system may be overtaxed. Consult a certified electrician for questions or concerns. Inspect wires, and immediately discontinue using any appliances with frayed or exposed wiring.

165. How can grease fires and burns be prevented in the kitchen?
Avoid grease build-up in the kitchen and on appliances. Do not leave unattended food cooking on stovetops; use back burners; and keep pot handles turned toward the back of the stove where children cannot reach them. If a fire occurs, smother it with a pot/pan lid or a cookie sheet, or close the oven door and turn off the source of heat. Do not store flammable or combustible items near the stove, including pot holders, towels, and aprons. Such items should be stored at least 3 feet away from heat sources.

166. Are some space heaters safer than others?
Yes. Make sure that a space heater will automatically shut off if it is tipped over. Consult the manufacturer's instructions to make sure that you use the heater as the manufacturer intended. When using open-space heaters or cooking near fireplaces, avoid wearing loose fitting clothes, which can catch fire easier than short or more fitted clothing.

167. Why should children never be put to sleep in day wear?
Fire-retardant sleepwear can make a difference in burn outcomes. Children should not sleep in loose fitting T-shirts or other oversized clothes made from cotton blends, which can catch fire easily. Look for clothing made from 100% polyester, which is flame-resistant and does not require chemical treatment. Clothing should be snug fitting. Short or more fitted clothing is less apt to catch fire.

WATER SAFETY

168. What key points should be noted about a life jacket, or personal flotation device (PFD)?
- All children should wear life jackets when boating or on the water. Federal law requires recreational boaters to carry a Coast Guard-approved life jacket of the correct size and in good condition for each person aboard a vessel in U.S. waters.
- A newer Coast Guard regulation requires that wearable life jackets be provided for people on boats less than 16 feet in length. Substituting throwable, type IV cushions for wearable life jackets is no longer permitted.

- Compliance with state and local life jacket ordinances is mandatory. Many states require PFDs for children up to age 12 at all times when on the water. Be sure to know what the laws of your area or providence require.
- The buoyancy and life-saving value of life jacket decrease over time. Drying a life jacket in a dryer, in front of a radiator, or with other source of direct heat destroys its buoyancy.

169. How can I be sure a particular life jacket is right for me?
- Follow the recommendations and guidelines for each of the five types of flotation devices. You should choose your PFD based on boating activities and conditions.
- Buy a PFD that you will wear, remembering that rescuers see bright colors more easily.
- Try on the jacket, and learn how to adjust it for a snug fit. After purchase, test it in the water. Make sure that it supports you and keeps your mouth and head clear of the water with no effort on your part. Then try pulling it on in the water—it is not as easy as it seems!

170. What should parents know about children wearing PFDs?
A life jacket is no substitute for adult supervision of children in and around the water. Children float differently than adults. Because their body weight is distributed differently, children are more likely to float face down in the water.

171. Do swimming lessons or a PFD make a child "water-safe"?
No. Children still need to follow water safety rules and should always swim with an adult.

172. What safety rules about diving into water should children be taught and reminded of frequently?
In addition to general water safety rules, a child should never jump or dive into any body of water unless the lifeguard or an adult says that it is safe. Jump in the deep end of a pool, and avoid diving, unless it is a pool designed for diving (usually deeper than 12 feet or 4 meters). When swimming in a new place, wade into the water feet first—never jump or dive. Do not dive off piers, docks, or rocks. Always raise your hands over your head when diving, and never let your friends dare you into diving.

173. For every drowning death in children, about how many children are hospitalized for near-drowning?
According to the National SAFE KIDS campaign, for every child that drowns, an additional four are hospitalized for near-drowning. Fifteen percent of children admitted for near drowning die in the hospital.

174. What common levels of protection are used to enhance the safety of a pool area?
- Yard fencing
- Pool fencing
- Child personal flotation devices
- Rope and float line
- Shepherd's hook
- Pool-side phone
- Posted safety information such as instructions for cardiopulmonary resuscitation and rescue breathing

Recent changes in law that may affect new construction in your area:
- Pool covers: mesh fences now must have one pole permanently attached to the home or deck.
- Alarms for pool gates, windows, doors, or the pool surface must be hard-wired to an electrical source.
- New drain system requirements prevent swimmers from being trapped.

Check local statutes and ordinances to be sure.

175. How is a shepherd's hook made useful for pulling someone to safety?
Affix the simple hook to an extension pole. People often neglect to attach a shepherd's hook to a pole, making it useless in an emergency when someone needs to be pulled to safety from a short distance.

176. What steps can be taken to make backyard pools safer?
- Installation of barriers: a four-sided fence, at least 4 feet or higher, with a self-closing, self-latching gate. The latch must be out of a child's reach.
- Supervision: nothing can replace adult supervision. Always watch children in the water. Someone should be assigned to watch children at a pool gathering. Never assume that someone else is watching your children.
- Enforcement of safety rules: no running around the pool, no glass in the pool area, no horseplay in and around the pool area.
- Preparation for emergencies: a cordless phone, emergency numbers, first-aid kit, and rescue equipment should be kept at or near the pool. Learn cardiopulmonary resuscitation, rescue breathing, and first aid.

177. Are thrashing around, coughing, and sputtering associated with drowning children?
No. Children drown very quickly and relatively silently.

178. Can inflatable wing-like floatation devices be used in place of PFDs?
Inflatable toys and wing-like floatation devices are not considered life-saving devices. Inflatable toys should never be considered a replacement for an age-appropriate, U.S. Coast Guard-approved PFD or adult supervision of children.

179. Are any PFDs considered appropriate for use in swimming pools?
According to the National Safety Council, a child who cannot swim should start with a U.S. Coast Guard-approved type II PFD. When the child has more control in the water (e.g., the ability to turn onto his or her back), move to a U.S. Coast Guard-approved type III PFD.

180. When should swimmers leave the pool or body of water during inclement weather?
The American Red Cross advises swimmers to exit the pool when they see storm clouds or hear thunder.

181. What is the second leading cause of unintentional injury-related death in children aged 1–14 years in the United States?
Drowning.

182. Why are barriers necessary around the pool?
Barriers are not childproof, but they provide layers of protection for a child who strays from supervision. Barriers give an adult additional time to locate a child before the unexpected becomes a reality.

183. What can be done to help in a drowning situation?
If someone is drowning and is within reach, grab an extension, such as a pole, for the person to hold onto. If the person is out of reach, throw a lifesaver with a rope attached to it, and try to pull the person to safety. If you must enter the water to help someone, take along an additional type of flotation (even a foam pool noodle) to assist you in case the person's thrashing puts you at risk of drowning. Look for signs of breathing and consciousness. Rescue breathing and cardiopulmonary resuscitation should be used as necessary. Even without formal training, you can still open the airway and breathe for the person.

184. What advice can be given to swimmers who find themselves in a rip current?
Do not try to fight the strong flow of rip currents and undertows, and do not panic. Ride with the flow of the water until you are able to catch your breath and get your bearings. Swim

calmly and smoothly parallel to the shore until you are no longer being pulled outward. Then swim to shore.

185. What simple procedure reduces the risk of injury and drowning?

Swimming with a partner or group and avoiding the use of alcohol dramatically reduce the risk of injury and drowning.

FIREARM SAFETY

186. What mistakes in judgment do parents often make in regard to children and firearms?

According to the National SAFE KIDS campaign, parents commonly have unrealistic perceptions of a child's capabilities and behavior regarding guns and misunderstand a child's ability to access and fire a gun. In addition, parents often believe that a child can distinguish between a real and a toy gun, will make good judgments about handling a gun, and will consistently follow rules about gun safety.

187. What should parents do to protect their children from firearms kept in the home?

Always store a firearm in a locked area, such as a safe, vault, or cabinet, or with a trigger-locking mechanism (metal, not plastic) in place. Do not place a trigger lock on a loaded gun; it can still discharge with the lock in place. Store the ammunition separately in a locked location. Ensure that children do not have access to the keys.

188. What issues can parents discuss with their children to make real the dangers of firearms?

Talk to your children about what to do if they find a gun, and explain that what they see on television and in movies when people fire guns is not real. In real life, guns hurt and kill people. Teach children the difference between toy and real guns. Before age 8 years children often cannot tell the difference between a real and a toy gun, nor do they understand the consequences of using a gun. However, children as young as 3 years of age have the strength to pull the trigger of many handguns.

189. Should parents talk about their child's safety and firearms with anyone outside the home?

Yes. Parents and caregivers should talk to the adults of any home that the child may visit (neighbors, baby sitters, friends, relatives) to find out if they own a gun and how they store it. Almost half of the homes in America contain firearms. A little investigative work on the parent's part can save a lifetime of grief.

190. For every child killed with a gun, how many more children are injured?

The Centers for Disease Control and Prevention report that for every child killed with a gun, four more children are injured. This reflects a mortality rate for children that is 12 times higher in the U.S. than in 25 other industrialized nations combined.

191. What should I tell my children to do if they find a gun and no adult is present?

Teach your children not to touch the gun and to call 911 or the local emergency number.

192. What important message can be communicated to the parent who keeps a firearm in the home for protection?

Guns kept in the home for protection are 22 times more likely to be used to kill a family member or friend than to kill in self-defense.

193. What other important risks are associated with the presence of a gun in the home?

The mere presence of a gun in the home increases the risk of domestic homicide by approximately threefold and the risk of suicide in the home by about fivefold.

BIBLIOGRAPHY

1. Centers for Disease Control and Prevention: Firearm Mortality and Morbidity. Atlanta, GA, Centers for Disease Control and Prevention, 1997.
2. Coffman S: Promotion of safety helmets for child bicyclists. Online Journal of Knowledge Synthesis Nursing, vol. 3, document no. 6, 1996.
3. Emergency Nurses Association: Trauma Nursing Core Course, 5th ed. Park Ridge, IL, Emergency Nurses Association, 2001.
4. Kellermann A, et al: Injuries and deaths due to firearms in the home. J Trauma Injury Infect Crit Care 45:263–267, 1998.
5. National Highway Transportation Safety Administration: Standardized Child Passenger Safety Training Program: Participant Manual, HS 366 R2/00. Washington, DC, National Highway Transportation Safety Administration, 2000.
6. National Highway Transportation Safety Administration: Traffic Safety Facts, 1999. Washington, DC, National Highway Transportation Safety Administration, 1999.
7. Smiley Holtzman D: The Panic Proof Parent: Creating a Safe Lifestyle for Your Family. Chicago, Contemporary Books, 2000.

Websites

AAA Foundation for Traffic Safety: www.aaafts.org/
American Academy of Pediatrics: www.aap.org/
Americans For Gun Safety: http://ww2.americansforgunsafety.com
American Society of Mechanical Engineers: www.asme.org
Association for the Advancement of Automotive Medicine: www.carcrash.org
American Public Health Association: http://wwwlapha.org/
Injury Control and Emergency Health Services Section of APHA: http://www.injurycontrol.com/ICEHS
American Trauma Society: www.amtrauma.org
Bicycle Federation of America: www.bikefed.org
Bicycle helmet data: http://rmstewart.uthsca.edu/fatalbrain/helmet.html
Bicycle Helmet Safety Institution (fact sheets): www.bhsi.org
Boating safety: www.boatus.com or www.floridaconservation.org
Brain Injury Association: www.biausa.org
Buckle Up America: www.buckleupamerica.org
Cease Fire: www.ceasefire.org (firearm safety)
Center for Injury Prevention: www.cipsafe.org
Children's Safety Network: http://www.edc.org/hhd/csn/
CSN National Injury and Violence Prevention Resource Center: http://www.edc.org/HHD/csn
Child Passenger Safety ListServe: www.CPSPList@yahoogroups.com
Child restraint recall list available from the NHTSA website: www.nhtsa.dot.gov/people/injury/childps/recall/cannister.htm
Community Preventive Services: http://web.health.gov/communityguide/
Consumer Advisory, October, 1999, Transportation Tips, 1998 www.nhtsa.dot.gov
Consumer Product Safety Commission: www.cpsc.gov/
ListServer (copies of product recall and product safety information can be sent automatically, as released by CPSC) to subscribe, send an e-mail message to listproc@cpsc.gov. In the message area, enter: join CSPCINFO-L.
Emergency Nurses Association: www.ena.org
Farm Safety 4 Just Kids: http://www.fs4jk.org
Firearm safety: http://depts.washington.edu/hiprc/childinjury/topic/firearms
Health Information Database: http://nhic-nt.health.org/newsrch.htm
Insurance Institute for Highway Safety (safety/fatalityfacts): www.iihs.org
National Children's Center for Rural and Agricultural Health and Safety: www.marshmed.org/nfmc/children/
National Child Passenger Safety Board: www.cpsboard.org
National Council on Alcoholism and Drug Dependence: http://www.ncaad.org
National Council on Firework Safety, Inc.: www.fireworksafety.com
National Health Information Resource Center: http://www.nhirc.org
National Highway Traffic Safety Administration (NHTSA): http://www.nhtsa.dot.gov/
National Institute on Drug Abuse: http://www.nida.nih.gov/
National Program for Playground Safety: www.uni.edu/playgrund/
National SAFE KIDS Campaign (safety tips): www.safekids.org
National Safety Belt Coalition: (202) 296-6263
National Safety Council (fact sheet library): www.nsc.org/

National Transportation Safety Board: www.ntsb.gov/
National Youth Sports Foundation: www.nyssf.org
Pool & Spa Living Magazine review of safety oriented products: www.poolspaliving.com
Pyschoactive durg information: www.erowid.org
Safe Ride News: www.saferide@twbc.com
Safety- Belt Safe U.S.A.: www.carseat.org
Society of Automotive Engineers: www.sae.org
Think First (brain injury prevention program): www.thinkfirst.org
U.S. Census Bureau: http://www.census.gov/
U.S. Centers for Disease Control and Prevention: http://www.cdc.gov and Morbidity and Mortality
      Weekly Report: http://www.cdc.gov/epo/mmwr/mmwr.html
U.S. Department of Health and Human Services: http://www.os.dhhs.gov
U.S. Fire Administration: www.usfa.fema.gov/
U.S. National Center for Health Statistics: http://www.cdc.gov/nchswww/default.htm
U.S. National Institutes of Health (NIH): http://www.nih.gov/welcome/
U.S. NIH Guide for Grants and Contracts (funding opportunities): http://www.nih.gov/grants/guide/
      index.html
World Health Organization: http://www.who.int/
Free access to Medline: http://www.nlm.nih.gov/databases/freemedl.html

Trauma-related websites
www.facs.org/fellows_info/other_sites/wbsttrauma.html
www.healthlinkusa.com
www.humc.edu/trauma/trmalink.htm
www.nscot.org/links.htm
www.trauma.org/resources/guide-web.html
www.traumanurse.org

III. System Injuries

7. HEAD AND NECK TRAUMA

Karen March, RN, MN, CNRN, CCRN

ACUTE BRAIN INJURY

1. What are the most common injuries to the head and neck?

Scalp lacerations, traumatic brain injury (TBI), facial fractures, traumatic cerebrovascular injuries, spinal fractures, and spinal cord injuries.

2. What is the difference between a primary and secondary injury?

The **primary injury** occurs at the time of injury or impact. The **secondary injury** results from subsequent events that affect oxygenation and perfusion of the brain tissue.

3. What mechanisms result in TBI?

MECHANISM	DEFINITION	EXAMPLES
Acceleration	Moving object hits a stationary head	Baseball, fist, hammer
Deceleration	Moving head hits a stationary object	Windshield, wall, ground
Acceleration-deceleration	Moving object comes to an abrupt stop	High-speed motor vehicle crashes, vehicle vs. pedestrian crashes
Coup-contrecoup	Results from movement of the intracranial contents within the cranium; the brain first hits the wall of cranium (coup), then bounces in the opposite direction and hits the cranium directly opposite the initial impact (contrecoup)	Falls, hitting the windshield
Penetrating	Object enters the skull and injures the brain	Knives, scissors, gunshot

4. What are the two types of primary brain injuries?

Injuries to the brain may be focal or diffuse. A **focal** brain injury produces a macroscopic lesion, such as scalp lacerations, skull fractures, lacerations and contusions of the brain, extradural hematomas (EDHs), subdural hematomas (SDHs), and intracerebral hematomas (ICHs). A **diffuse** brain injury is microscopic or neuronal; examples include concussion and diffuse axonal injury.

5. What are the three types of skull fractures?

1. Linear: a crack in the skull.
2. Depressed: the bone is depressed more than half the width of the skull.
3. Basilar: linear fracture in the base of the skull.

6. What are the signs and symptoms of a basilar skull fracture?

Fractures in the anterior fossa: periorbital ecchymosis (raccoon or panda eyes) and blood or cerebral spinal fluid (CSF) drainage from the nose (rhinorrhea).

Fractures in the middle or posterior fossa: bruising over the mastoid process (Battle sign) and blood and CSF drainage from the ear (otorrhea).

7. How are basilar skull fractures managed?

Assess for the presence of CSF drainage from the nose or mouth either by testing the drainage fluid for glucose with a Dextrostix or, if blood is present, by performing a halo ring test. The halo ring test is performed by placing a few drops of CSF on a pillow case or paper towel. Blood congeals in the center, and the CSF forms a ring around it. Avoid packing the nose or ear when a CSF leak is present. Packing obstructs the flow of CSF and increases the risk of infections. Patients with rhinorrhea or otorrhea may be treated with antibiotics. Most CSF leaks seal themselves after several days of bedrest with the head of the bed elevated. A lumbar or ventricular drain may be inserted to lower the CSF pressure against the tear. Surgery is reserved for larger defects or defects that do not heal spontaneously.

8. What is the difference between laceration and contusion of the brain? In what parts of the brain do such injuries most often occur?

A **laceration** is the tearing of the brain that occurs when the brain impacts the rough undersurface of the basal cranium or results from a depressed skull fracture. A **contusion** is the bruising of the cortical surfaces of the brain. Lacerations and contusions of brain tissue are usually found in the frontal and temporal lobes.

9. How do epidural (extradural) hematomas and subdural hematomas differ?

EDHs are hemorrhages that occur between the skull and the dura and are often associated with a linear skull fracture, which lacerates the middle meningeal artery. An **SDH** is a hemorrhage caused by tearing of the bridging veins or small arteries over the surface of the brain, forming a hematoma between the dura and the brain.

10. Why is an EDH called the "talk and die syndrome?"

Patients often have a lucid period immediately after they are injured before they deteriorate and die. Death results from rapid expansion of the hematoma, which causes uncal herniation.

11. Describe the three types of SDHs and how they are managed.

Acute SDH is symptomatic in the first 24–72 hours after injury and usually requires immediate surgical evacuation.

Subacute SDH is symptomatic 72 hours to two weeks after injury and is managed by close observation for symptoms of increased intracranial pressure and herniation. Surgery is usually avoided because of the consistency of the clot, which is allowed to reabsorb.

Chronic SDH exhibits symptoms 2 weeks or more after injury and mimics dementia. Chronic SDH is seen most often in elderly patients or chronic substance abusers with brain atrophy. Bleeding is slow, and more space is available for expansion of the clot before the patient deteriorates neurologically. Treatment consists of burr holes, irrigation, and insertion of catheters to drain the clot slowly. Patients are nursed in the supine position to promote drainage and to avoid reaccumulation of the clot. Keeping the head supine allows the brain tissue to expand and take up the space in the cranium previously occupied by the clot.

12. How is an intracerebral hematoma different from other intracranial hematomas?

An ICH is bleeding into the brain parenchyma. Surgery is avoided unless the clot is large and causes a mass effect because surgery requires removal of brain tissue.

13. Why do gunshot wounds to the head carry such a high mortality rate?

The morbidity and mortality from gunshot wounds to the head depend on the type of weapon, shape and trajectory of the bullet, structures hit by the bullet, and whether the bullet crosses the midline. In general, transventricular gunshot wounds are fatal (overall mortality rate of 50–60%). Bullets cause not only direct injury to the tissues in their path but also indirect injury to surrounding tissue as a result of the cavitation from the velocity and yaw of the bullet.

14. What is the difference between concussion and diffuse axonal brain injury?
Concussions and diffuse axonal brain injuries are microscopic or cellular injuries. A cerebral **concussion** is defined as a temporary loss of consciousness, usually for less than 6 hours, with no long-term neurologic sequelae. **Diffuse axonal injuries** (DAIs), also called shearing or Stritch injuries, result from damage to cell axons and activation of a biochemical process that further destroys these axons. DAI produces prolonged coma and carries significant morbidity and mortality.

15. Explain the "storming" or autonomic dysfunction syndrome that frequently occurs after DAI.
Autonomic dysfunction syndrome or "storming" (also called diencephalic seizures) is a set of symptoms resulting from a dysfunction of sympathetic regulation that produces increased intracranial pressure (ICP), dilated pupils, diaphoresis, hypertension, and abnormal flexion or extensor posturing. These symptoms diminish with time and may be moderated with use of propranolol, morphine sulfate, and bromocriptine.

16. What is traumatic subarachnoid hemorrhage?
Traumatic subarachnoid hemorrhage is bleeding into the subarachnoid space, which occurs in 30–40% of TBIs and puts the patient at risk for developing cerebral vasospasm. Vasospasm is the narrowing of the vessel lumen that may result in a delayed ischemic event. The risk for developing vasospasm is highest 3–5 days after the bleeding.

17. What is mild TBI?
The patient with a mild TBI may have a normal CT scan and may or may not have a loss of consciousness. The Glasgow Coma Scale (GCS) score is 13–15. Deficits become apparent only after the patient tries to resume normal activities. Symptoms include somatic, cognitive, and emotional disturbances. Sequelae from an untreated mild TBI may result in loss of employment and disruption of the family.

18. What are the symptoms of mild TBI?

SOMATIC	COGNITIVE	EMOTIONAL-BEHAVIORAL
Headache	Amnesia of event	Agitation
Dizziness	Impaired attention and concen-	Irritability
Nausea and vomiting	tration	Apathy
Blurred vision	Impaired short-term memory	Depression
Tinnitus and hearing	Disorientation and/or confusion	Emotional instability
difficulties	Slow thinking and information	Sleep disturbance
Drowsiness	processing	Lower tolerance for frustration
Seizures (rare)	Poor judgment	Loss of sexual drive
	Mental fatigue	Intolerance to alcohol

19. What is the treatment for mild TBI?
Education of patient and family about coping strategies and acknowledgment that symptoms are real can help the patient get through this period. Symptoms are usually self-limiting.

20. What is secondary brain injury?
Secondary brain injury results from the biochemical and biophysical processes that lead to further injury and cell death. To minimize secondary injury, we must monitor and treat systemic and intracranial processes that may result in secondary injury.

SYSTEMIC PROCESSES	INTRACRANIAL PROCESSES
Hypoxia	Intracranial hypertension
Hypotension	Delayed intracerebral hemorrhage
Electrolyte imbalance	Edema
Anemia	Hyperemia
Hyperthermia	Carotid dissection
Hypercarbia	Seizures
Hypoglycemia	Vasospasm

21. What is intracranial compliance?

Intracranial compliance is the ability to adapt to increases in intracranial volume, blood, brain tissue, or CSF by decreasing the other elements of volume (Monro-Kellie doctrine) to maintain a normal intracranial pressure (ICP). Normal mechanisms include shunting of CSF into the spinal canal and increasing venous outflow. When compliance is lost, intracranial pressure increases.

22. What are the neurologic signs of increased ICP?

Changes in level of consciousness, headache, nausea and vomiting, pupil changes (unilateral or bilateral dilated and nonreactive pupils), impaired extraocular movements, motor deficits, abnormal or absent brainstem reflexes (corneal, cough, gag), abnormal respirations, hypertension with a widening pulse pressure, and tachycardia or bradycardia.

23. What are the most common ways to monitor ICP?

- Ventricular catheter with external fluid-filled transducer or hybrid catheters (fiberoptic or internal strain-gauge transducers within the system)
- Parenchymal bolts (fiberoptic or internal strain-gauge transducers)
- Subdural catheters.

24. What is the normal configuration of an ICP waveform? What its significance?

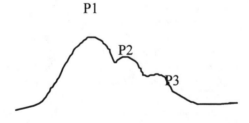

P1	P2	P3
Percussion wave	Tidal wave	Dicrotic wave
Reflects the ejection of blood from the heart transmitted through the choroid plexus in ventricles	Reflects brain bulk or compliance, vasomotor paralysis, swelling and edema	Aortic valve closure
	Reflects venous compartment	
	P2 = 80% P1	

As P2 becomes equal to or greater than P1, compliance is lost and ICP becomes elevated within the next 24 hours.

25. What are A, B, and C waves?

A, B, and C waves are trends in ICP. C is the normal fluctuation in ICP. B waves are short spikes in ICP that start from a slight elevation in ICP but are not sustained. A waves or plateau waves are ICP elevations that are sustained for 20–30 minutes and can exceed 100 mmHg.

26. What is normal ICP?

0–10 mmHg.

27. What are the Brain Trauma Guidelines?

These evidence-based recommendations for the management of severe TBI were first released in 1995 and revised in 2000.

TOPIC	RECOMMENDATION
Trauma system	*Guideline:* All regions in the U.S. should have a trauma system. *Option:* Neurosurgeons should have organized approach to care.
Initial management	*Option:* First priority of treatment is complete fluid resuscitation. Do not treat ICP unless signs of herniation are present.
Resuscitation of blood pressure and oxygen	*Guideline:* Avoid hypotension (systolic blood pressure < 90 mmHg), hypoxia (PaO_2 < 60 mmHg). *Option:* Maintain mean systemic arterial blood pressure ≥ 90 mmHg
Indications for monitoring of intracranial pressure (ICP)	*Guideline:* ICP monitoring recommended for patients with: 1. GCS score of 3–8 with abnormal computed tomography (CT) scan 2. Normal CT with two or more of the following: • Age > 40 years • Motor posturing • Blood pressure < 90 mmHg 3. GCS score of 9–15 with abnormal CT (at physician's discretion)
ICP treatment threshold	*Guideline:* ICP should be treated at 20–25 mmHg. *Option:* Corroborate ICP by clinical exam before treatment.
Cerebral perfusion pressure (CPP)	*Option:* CCP should be maintained at a minimum of 70 mmHg in adults.
Hyperventilation	*Standard:* Chronic prolonged hyperventilation ($PaCO_2$ of 25 mmHg) should be avoided in the absence of increased ICP. *Guideline:* Prophylactic hyperventilation ($PaCO_2$ ≤ 35 mmHg) should be avoided during the first 24 hours. *Option:* Brief hyperventilation may be used to treat acute neurologic deterioration or refractory increased ICP.
Mannitol	*Guideline:* Mannitol is effective in treating ICP and should be given as a bolus of 0.25–1 gm/kg of body weight. *Option:* Use of mannitol before ICP monitoring is indicated with signs of herniation or neurologic deterioration. Avoid hypovolemia. Keep serum osmolarity < 320 mOsm.
Barbiturates	*Guideline:* High-dose barbiturate therapy may be used in hemodynamically stable patients refractory to other ICP treatments.
Steroids	*Standard:* Steroids are not recommended.
Nutrition	*Guideline:* Nutritional replacement of 140% of resting metabolism in nonparalyzed patients and 100% in paralyzed patients using enteral or parenteral feedings by 7 days.
Seizure treatment	*Standard:* Prophylactic use of anticonvulsants is not recommended to prevent late posttraumatic seizures. *Option:* Early posttraumatic seizures may or may not be treated; no effect on outcome.

PaO_2 = partial arterial oxygen tension, $PaCO_2$ = partial pressure of carbon dioxide in arterial blood.

28. What are the current treatments for severe TBI?

TREATMENT	ADDITIONAL INFORMATION
Fluid resuscitation	Euvolemia achieved with isotonic solution (normal saline, lactated Ringer's solution).
Avoid hypotension	Systolic blood pressure (SBP) < 90 mmHg doubles the mortality rate. Hypotension in infants and children is defined as SBP ≤ 50 percentile for age (about 65–70 mmHg for infants, 85 mmHg for adolescents).
Avoid aggressive treatment of hypertension	Blood pressure should not be treated unless it exceeds 220/130 mmHg or the patient shows signs of other organ dysfunction.
Maintain adequate cerebral perfusion pressure (CPP)	In adults, CPP should be maintained at about 70 mmHg. In children CPP should be adjusted to age-appropriate levels (70–80 percentile for age).
ICP treatment thresholds	ICP should be treated if > 20–25 mmHg in adults, > 10 mmHg in infants, and > 15 mmHg in small children.
Diuretic therapy	Mannitol bolus is recommend at 0.25–1 gm/kg. Care should be taken to avoid systemic dehydration. Maintain a serum osmolarity < 310–320 mOsm. Loop diuretic may also be used with care to maintain euvolemia.
Hyperventilation	For every millimeter change in $PaCO_2$ there is a 3% change in blood flow. Hyperventilation should be avoided during the first 24 hours after injury unless signs of acute herniation are present. $PaCO_2$ should be maintained at about 35 mmHg and hyperventilation increased with care. Aggressive hyperventilation should be instituted only when cerebral blood flow has been measured and is hyperemic (high).
Surgery	Surgery is recommended for mass lesions such as hematomas. Hemicraniectomy may be performed in patients with uncontrolled ICP.
Cerebrospinal fluid (CSF) drainage	Ventricular drainage of CSF may be used to control ICP. Small amounts of drainage by continuous or intermittent methods.
Anticonvulsants	Anticonvulsants in the immediate postinjury period have been shown to prevent early posttraumatic seizures but do not improve outcome. Long-term seizure prophylaxis is not recommended unless seizures occur.
Positioning	Keep head in a neutral alignment to promote jugular venous outflow. Elevation of head of bed by 30° is recommended by most, but the position should be based on hemodynamic stability and individual response.
Sedation	Pain management and sedation are used to decrease metabolic demand. Barbiturates and propofol may be used to induce coma, thereby decreasing metabolism and blood flow and decreasing ICP. Patients should be hemodynamically stable before administration of drugs.
Glucose	Avoid hypo- and hyperglycemia. Glucose > 200–250 mg/dl increases morbidity and mortality.
Temperature	Maintain normothermia. Hyperthermia increases metabolic demand and may worsen outcome. Hypothermia has not been shown to improve outcome.

$PaCO_2$ = partial pressure of carbon dioxide in arterial blood.

29. What are the common complications of TBI? How are they treated?

COMPLICATION	TREATMENT
Pulmonary: pneumonia and atelectasis	Patients require meticulous pulmonary toilet and aspiration precautions. When suctioning, hyperoxygenate and hyperinflate but do not hyperventilate. Premedication with sedation or lidocaine before suctioning may minimize effects on intracranial pressure.
Seizures	Seizure precautions
Deep vein thrombosis (DVT)	Prophylaxis: antiembolic stockings, sequential compression devices, anticoagulation
Contractures/spasticity	Range-of-motion exercises, positioning for function, splints, antispasmodic drugs
Dysphagia	Swallowing evaluation and modified diet or alternative feeding method (enteral or parenteral feeding)
Fluid and electrolyte	Diabetes insipidus: fluid replacement, antidiuretic hormone
	Syndrome of inappropriate antidiuretic hormone (SIADH): fluid restriction, sodium replacement (hypertonic, if severe), diuretic
	Cerebral salt-wasting: sodium replacement without restriction of fluids

30. What are the signs and symptoms of the common causes of fluid and electrolyte imbalance?

DIABETES INSIPIDUS	SIADH	CEREBRAL SALT-WASTING
Hypernatremia (> 145)	Hyponatremia (dilutional)	Hyponatremia (primary)
Hyperosmolarity (> 295)	↑ Extracellular fluid	↓ Extracellular fluid
Urine osmolarity < 300	Serum hypo-osmolarity (< 280)	Serum hypo-osmolarity (< 280)
Specific gravity < 1.005	↑ Plasma volume	↓ Plasma volume
Dehydration	↑ Body weight	↓ Body weight
	Low blood urea nitrogen	High blood urea nitrogen
	Not necessarily a negative salt balance	Excessive natriuresis
	Urine osmolarity is inappropriately concentrated compared with serum osmolarity	Negative salt balance (primary loss of sodium)

SIADH = syndrome of inappropriate antidiuretic hormone.

31. What is the Rancho scale? How is it used?

The Rancho (Rancho Los Amigos) scale is an assessment tool used to evaluate the recovery of brain-injured patients and to outline rehabilitation interventions.

LEVEL	DESCRIPTION	ASSESSMENT FINDINGS	INTERVENTIONS
Rancho 1	Coma (GCS 3)	No response	Sensory stimulation
Rancho 2	Generalized response	Posturing to withdrawal	Sensory stimulation
Rancho 3	Localized response	Withdrawal to localized response	Sensory stimulation
		Focuses and tracks	One-step commands
		Periods of alertness	Yes–no questions
		Spontaneous purposeful movements	Reorient
		Follows some one-step commands	

Table continued on following page

LEVEL	DESCRIPTION	ASSESSMENT FINDINGS	INTERVENTIONS
Rancho 4	Agitated and confused	Follows commands inconsistently Attempts communication Resists treatment Behavioral issues	Establish calm environment Manage behavior Reorient Encourage independent activities of daily living (ADLs) Limit choices
Rancho 5	Confused/inappropriate	Alert but confused Obeys simple commands	Reorient Encourage independent ADLs Assess learning carryover Safety
Rancho 6	Confused/appropriate	Oriented at times Follows commands	Provide structural environment Memory book Cueing Safety
Rancho 7	Automatic/appropriate	Minimal confusion Slowed learning	Increased independence Safety Community reintegration Vocational skills
Rancho 8	Purposeful/appropriate	Oriented	Complex tasks Vocational skills

MAXILLOFACIAL TRAUMA

32. What are the symptoms of facial injury?
Airway compromise, pain, tenderness or step-off of the face on palpation, bleeding, malocclusion of the teeth, facial asymmetry, cerebral spinal fluid (CSF) leakage from nose or ears.

33. List the most common types of facial fractures along with signs and symptoms and management strategies.

TYPE OF FRACTURE	SIGNS AND SYMPTOMS	TREATMENT
Zygomatic (tripod)	Step-off defect, periorbital ecchymosis, subconjunctival hemorrhage, facial edema, upward gaze, enophthalmos (sunken eye), trismus (inability to open mouth), infraorbital hyperesthesia, diplopia, epistaxis, possible rhinorrhea, asymmetry of face	Maintain airway, elevation of head of bed if cervical spine is cleared, cold pack to face, possible surgery
Mandible fracture	Airway compromise, malocclusion of teeth, facial asymmetry, pain with jaw movement or palpation, trismus, palpable fracture, dental injury about canine and third molar area, anesthesia of lower lip, ruptured tympanic membrane	Maintain airway, cold pack to face, immobilize with Barton dressing (bulky wrap around head), surgical fixation

Table continued on following page

TYPE OF FRACTURE	SIGNS AND SYMPTOMS	TREATMENT
Le Fort I (horizontal fracture through maxilla at level of nasal floor)	Epistaxis, lip laceration or fracture of teeth, malocclusion of teeth, mobile maxilla on palpation	Maintain airway, cold pack to face, surgical fixation
Le Fort II (pyramid-shaped fracture of midface involving superior nasal area)	Nose moves with dental arch with manipulation, nasal fracture with epistaxis, periorbital ecchymosis, subconjunctival ecchymosis, widening between eyes, rhinorrhea	Maintain airway (usually intubated), cold pack to face, surgical fixation, antibiotics
Le Fort III (total craniofacial separation)	Flattening and elongation of face, malocclusion, significant bleeding, edema and ecchymosis, front of face moves when dental arch manipulated, possible rhinorrhea, diplopia	Maintain airway (intubated), cold pack to face, surgical fixation, antibiotics
Orbital fracture	Diplopia, loss of vision, impaired extraocular movements, subconjuctival hemorrhage, enophthalmos, infraorbital pain or anesthesia, bony deformity	Ice pack, patch affected eye, consider antibiotics, surgical repair of fractures, monitor visual acuity

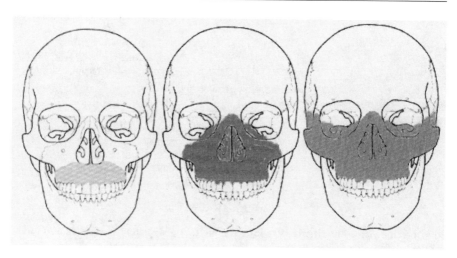

Left, Le Fort I fracture; *Center,* Le Fort 2 fracture; *Right,* Le Fort 3 fracture.

EARS, NOSE, AND THROAT TRAUMA

34. What are the common injuries to the ear?

TYPE OF INJURY	ASSESSMENT	THERAPEUTIC INTERVENTIONS
Simple laceration	Observe bleeding from ear	Irrigate wound Suture Topical antibiotic Administer tetanus

Table continued on following page

TYPE OF INJURY	ASSESSMENT	THERAPEUTIC INTERVENTIONS
Hematoma of pinna	Visible hematoma	Aspirate hematoma; drain may be inserted Small pressure dressing
Traumatic amputation of ear	Visible amputation	Reattach ear Administer antibiotics Administer tetanus
Thermal injury to ear	Visible burn or frostbite	Burn: wound care Frostbite: rewarm with moist heat (40°C)

35. Describe the most common injuries to the nose and their treatment.

TYPE OF INJURY	ASSESSMENT	THERAPEUTIC INTERVENTIONS
Epistaxis	Bleeding Deformity of the nose	Attention to airway, breathing, circulation (ABCs), particularly airway clearance Anterior bleeding • Slightly hyperextend neck • Suction clot • Identify site of bleeding and apply vasoconstrictor agent (usually cocaine) • Cauterize Nasal packing Posterior bleeding requires packing
Nasal fractures	Observe for swelling and/or deformity Palpate for crepitus and/or fracture X-ray	Cold pack Splint Control bleeding Local anesthesia before fracture set Drain hematoma if present Pack Administer tetanus

OCULAR TRAUMA

36. Describe vision-threatening eye injuries, including signs and symptoms and interventions.

TYPE	SIGNS AND SYMPTOMS	TREATMENT
Chemical burns to eye (alkaline: ammonia, magnesium hydroxide; acid: sulfuric, hydrochloric, hydrofluoric, acetic)	Pain, corneal opacification, other chemical burns of surrounding structures	Irrigate affected eye using neutral solution (normal saline, lactated Ringer's), administer medications, shield eye
Hyphema (collection of blood in the anterior chamber)	Blood in anterior chamber, deep aching pain, diminished visual acuity, increased intraocular pressure	Shield eye, position with head or bed elevated, ophthalmologic consult

Table continued on following page

TYPE	SIGNS AND SYMPTOMS	TREATMENT
Global rupture or disruption (blunt or penetrating)	Loss or reduction of vision, pain, impaled object or global disruption, extrusion of aqueous or vitreous humor	Stabilize impaled object, shield globe, no medications to eye, prepare for surgery

37. Define traumatic optic neuritis. What are the symptoms? How is it treated?

Unilateral visual deterioration due to injury to the optic nerve, usually as a result of a blow to the head that causes bony deformity of the optic canal. Symptoms include an afferent pupil defect, loss of visual acuity, central scotoma, and retro-orbital pain. Treatment includes high-dose steroids and surgical decompression of the optic deformity.

NECK TRAUMA

38. What are the three zones of injuries to the neck?

ZONE	REGION	STRUCTURES AFFECTED
1	Clavicle to cricothyroid cartilage	Subclavian artery and vein
2	Cricothyroid cartilage to angle of mandible	Thyroid and parathyroid glands, common carotid, jugular vein, larynx, trachea
3	Angle of mandible to base of skull	Bifurcation of carotid: internal and external carotid arteries, upper jugular vein

39. What are the signs and symptoms of laryngotracheal injuries?
- Hoarseness
- Cough with hemoptysis
- Progressive stridor
- Respiratory distress
- Subcutaneous emphysema
- Pain and tenderness
- Flattened appearance of larynx

40. What is the treatment for laryngotracheal injuries?
- Intubation
- Cricothyroidotomy or tracheostomy
- High-flow oxygen
- Antibiotics
- Steroids (if indicated)
- Surgical repair
- Rest voice

41. What are the common causes of vascular injuries to the neck? What are the possible sequelae?

Injuries and common causes include penetrating injuries (gunshot and knife wounds) and blunt injuries (hyperextension or subluxation of spine, mandibular fractures). Sequelae of vascular injuries include transient ischemic attacks (TIAs) or stroke.

42. Describe the treatment for vascular injuries to the neck.

Direct pressure, anticoagulation, and revascularization.

SPINE TRAUMA

43. What are the anatomic elements of the spine?

Vertebrae, nucleus pulposus, ligaments, arterial blood supply, and spinal cord.

44. What mechanisms cause spine injuries? What types of injuries do they produce?

MECHANISM	TYPE OF INJURY
Hyperextension	Compression of posterior elements of vertebrae, disruption of anterior ligaments, central cord injury in elderly
Hyperflexion	Compression of anterior elements of vertebrae (body), disruption of posterior ligaments, possible anterior spinal artery injury
Rotation	Disruption of multiple ligaments, facet dislocation, severe spinal cord injuries
Loading or compression	Dispersion of energy along spine producing multiple spine fractures and multiple levels of injury

45. Distinguish between complete and incomplete spinal cord injury.

A **complete** injury is loss of all sensory, motor, and reflex function below the level of the injury. An **incomplete** injury has some preservation of sensory or motor function.

46. What are the four commonly described incomplete spinal cord injuries?

1. **Anterior cord syndrome** involves deficits of the corticospinal and spinothalamic tracts with preservation of the posterior columns.

2. **Central cord syndrome** deficits are greater in the upper than lower extremities.

3. **Brown-Sequard syndrome** involves ipsilateral loss of motor and proprioception with contralateral loss of pain and temperature sensation.

4. **Posterior column syndrome** involves loss of proprioception, light touch, and vibration.

47. What is the difference between spinal shock and neurogenic shock?

Spinal shock is the loss of all sensory, motor, and reflex activity below the level of injury. It occurs within minutes and is usually seen in lesions above T6. Spinal shock may last for days or months.

Disruption in sympathetic nervous system function often occurs, resulting in neurogenic shock. Poikilothermia, the loss of temperature control, may occur in injuries at the level of T1 or above. **Neurogenic shock** is characterized by ineffective circulating volume, which results in inadequate organ and tissue perfusion due to loss of sympathetic innervation. It is seen most commonly with injuries at C3–C5 but may be seen at T1 or above. Symptoms include hypotension (rarely < 70 mmHg), bradycardia, decreased respirations, decreased urine output, decreased mental status, and warm, flushed, dry skin. Treatment includes the modified Trendelenburg position, fluid resuscitation, and alpha-adrenergic vasoconstricting drugs (e.g., phenylephrine).

48. Describe the initial management of spinal cord injury.

Initial management includes the ABCs (airway, breathing, circulation), spine immobilization with a backboard and cervical collar, and administration of steroids (methylprednisolone, 30 mg/kg of body weight followed by 5.4 mg/kg for the next 24 or 48 hours). In the emergency department, spinal x-rays are performed to assess the extent of the injuries and determine whether other radiologic studies, such as computed tomography (CT) or magnetic resonance imaging (MRI), are needed. Cervical traction may be applied to further stabilize and align the cervical spine.

49. What should nurses keep in mind when administering methylprednisolone to patients with spinal cord injury?

1. Administer the 30 mg/kg over 15 minutes; 45 minutes later, administer the 5.4 mg/kg for either 24 hours (if begun before 3 hours) or 48 hours (if begun 3–8 hours after injury).

2. Contraindications include diabetes mellitus or other metabolic diseases, pregnancy, and penetrating injury.

3. Side effects include increased infection rates, particularly pneumonia and atelectasis, gastrointestinal bleeding, and hyperglycemia.

50. What methods are used for long-term stabilization of the spine?

Some patients undergo surgical stabilization with fusion, spine hardware, and external orthosis, whereas others can be stabilized simply with an external orthosis. External orthoses for the cervical spine include halo vests, cervical collars, Minerva vests, and other orthotics with cervical extensions.

51. How does a spinal cord injury affect the physiologic function of the body?

SYSTEM	NORMAL PHYSIOLOGY	FUNCTION AFTER INJURY
Pulmonary	*Pulmonary innervation* C1–C3: accessory muscles of neck C3–C5: diaphragm T2–T8: intercostal muscles T7–T12: abdominal muscles Inspiration: chest wall moves up and out, diaphragm flattens Expiration: recoil of chest wall Cough: requires deep breath and contraction of abdominal muscles	Cervical spine: vital capacity decreased by up to 58% Decreased tidal volume when abdominal and intercostal muscles impaired Protraction of chest with protrusion of abdomen Respiratory muscles initially flaccid, then spastic Postural dependency
Cardiac	Cardiac output = stroke volume × heart rate Total peripheral resistance: diameter of arteries Autonomic response mediated by medulla Cardiac center: heart rate Vasomotor center: peripheral vascular resistance Alpha-adrenergic receptors: vasoconstriction Beta-adrenergic receptors (myocardium): increase heart rate and contractility Stimulated by baroreceptors *Intravascular fluid volume* Antidiuretic hormone: water retention Renin-angiotensin-aldosterone: stimulates kidney to retain sodium and water *Cardiac innervation* Sympathetic innervation: preganglionic fibers at T1–T4 Parasympathetic (vagal nerve): originates in medulla	Ineffective circulating volume resulting in inadequate organ and tissue perfusion (neurogenic shock) Most common: C3–C5; but seen in T1 or above; may occur as low as T5 Autonomic dysreflexia: after spinal shock has subsided, noxious stimuli (e.g., full bladder or bowel, skin breakdown, bladder infections) may stimulate the sympathetic nervous system, resulting in vasoconstriction and hypertension. If hypertension is severe, patient may develop an intracranial hemorrhage. *Arrhythmias:* bradycardia, asystole Poikilothermia: impaired thermal regulation due to inability to constrict or dilate blood vessels in order to conserve heat or cool down
Musculoskeletal	*Corticospinal tract:* descends and crosses in the medulla *Upper motor neuron:* from brain to spinal cord Muscle weakness, spasticity, hyperreflexia, clonus	Spinal shock: areflexia, flaccidity, no sensation, loss of vasomotor tone Paralysis or paresis Spasticity: upper motor neuron injury Loss of brain moderation of reflex arcs

Table continued on following page

SYSTEM	NORMAL PHYSIOLOGY	FUNCTION AFTER INJURY
Musculoskeletal *(cont.)*	*Lower motor neuron:* from ventral root to muscle Flaccidity, atrophy, decreased reflexes, fasciculations	
Skin	Sensation: spinothalamic tract Lateral: pain and temperature Anterior: light touch Fibers cross in cord Prolonged pressure is sensed subconsciously and body position is adjusted to avoid the development of tissue ischemia and skin breakdown.	Altered sensation results in the inability to sense pain and pressure that signals the need to reposition the body weight, resulting in the build-up of excessive pressure (> 32 mmHg) and tissue ischemia.
Urinary	Parasympathetic innervation of bladder at S2–S4 mediates the contraction of the bladder needed to empty the bladder. Sympathetic innervation from T11 to L2 segments allows relaxation of the detrusor muscle and and closes the neck of the bladder, stopping micturition.	Initially the bladder may be flaccid, but spontaneous voiding may be initiated by tapping the suprapubic area in patients with supraspinal lesions after spinal shock has subsided. Hyperreflexic bladder (frequent contractions) is also seen in some cervical injuries, resulting in incontinence or difficulty in emptying the bladder.
Bowel	The sensation of a full rectum signaling the need to defecate is transmitted to the parasympathetic fibers at S2–S4, signaling the anus to relax. Sympathetic fibers originate from T8 to L3 and innervate the mucosa of the gastrointestinal tract, ileocecal sphincter, and the internal anal sphincter to contract.	Constipation Incontinence
Sexuality	Parasympathetic innervation: T11–12 causes vasodilatation of genitals and lubrication; activated by psychogenic stimuli. Sympathetic innervation (S2–S4) is activated by tactile stimulus. Sensory response to stimulus that triggers orgasm originates from T11–T12.	Ability to become aroused and have an orgasm may be possible, but the experience will be altered because of alterations in sensation. Sexual pleasure may be achieved by stimulation of different areas that become erotic.

52. What are the priorities of care after a cervical spine injury?

SYSTEM	INTERVENTIONS
Pulmonary	Goals: to prevent atelectasis and pneumonia Rotobed (before stabilization) Pulmonary toilet Assistive cough every 4 hours as needed for injuries at T10 and above

Table continued on following page

SYSTEM	INTERVENTIONS
Pulmonary *(cont.)*	Intermittent positive-pressure breathing as needed, every 4 hours.
	Incentive spirometry every 1–2 hours while awake with goal of ≥ 10 cc/kg body weight.
	Glossopharyngeal breathing: sequential gulps of air without expiration to build tidal volume.
	Mobilize patient out of bed.
Cardiovascular	Deep vein thrombosis
	Anticoagulation (enoxaparin, heparin)
	Antiembolism stockings/sequential compression devices
	Orthostasis
	Adequate hydration
	Ace wrap for legs (toes to groin)
	Ephedrine: alpha-adrenergic agent to raise systemic arterial blood pressure
	Altered temperature regulation: monitor environmental temperature to avoid hyperthermia or hypothermia.
	Autonomic dysreflexia: avoid noxious stimulation.
Musculoskeletal	Rotobed before spine is stabilized.
	Begin range-of-motion exercises.
	Measure for wheelchair.
	Out of bed at least twice daily; increase time daily (15 min/day) as tolerated.
	Pressure relief to prevent skin breakdown.
	Spasticity: antispasmodic (e.g., baclofen) if spasticity interferes with mobility.
Skin	Rotobed: rotate 20 of 24 hours per stabilization.
	Bed with pressure-reducing mattress after spine is stabilized.
	Avoid sitting up in bed to prevent shearing injuries.
	Pressure relief every 15 minutes while sitting.
	Inspect skin frequently.
	Start nutrition early.
Urinary	Foley catheter, intermittent catheterization, or spontaneous voiding. Some patients using the Crede maneuver of the suprapubic region or straining can initiate spontaneous voiding. Intermittent catheterization requires fluid restriction (1500–2000 cc/24 hour) to prevent overdistention of bladder.
	Medications may be used to facilitate bladder emptying or to increase tone.
Bowel	Bowel program: Ducolax with digital stimulation every 15 minutes up to 6 times. If no bowel movement in 24 hours, the addition of milk of magnesia or other medication to promote defecation should be used. A high-fiber diet is recommended to avoid constipation.
Psychosocial	Use rehabilitation psychology and spinal cord injury social worker to facilitate coping.
	Arrange patient and family care conferences.

BIBLIOGRAPHY

1. American Association of Neuroscience Nurses: AANN's Neuroscience Nursing: Human Responses to Neurologic Dysfunction. Philadelphia, W.B. Saunders. 2001.
2. Brain Trauma Foundation: Management and prognosis of severe traumatic brain injury. J Neurotrauma 17:453–627, 2000.
3. Bucher L, Melander S: Critical Care Nursing. Philadelphia, W.B. Saunders, 1999.
4. Cruz J: Neurologic and Neurosurgical Emergencies. Philadelphia, W.B. Saunders. 1998.
5. Emergency Nurses Association: Trauma Nursing Core Course, 5th ed. Chicago, Emergency Nurses Association, 2000.
6. Sheehy S, Blansfield J, Danis D, Gervasini A: Manual of Clinical Trauma Care: The First Hour. St. Louis, Mosby, 1999.
7. Tobias J: Traumatic brain injury in children: Initial resuscitation and ICU care. In Hyperbook of Neurosurgery. Columbia, MO, CyberMed LLC, 1998–2000.

8. THORACIC TRAUMA

Cindy Jimmerson, RN, and Steven D. Glow, RN, MSN, FNP, CEN, EMT-P

AIRWAY MANAGEMENT

1. Which types of chest injuries can compromise the airway?

Tracheal or bronchial injuries can disrupt the flow of air through the upper airway. Open ("sucking") chest wounds provide an alternative pathway for airflow. Air that leaks from either an injured lower airway or a sucking chest wound may make the airway inoperative if the diameter of the injury is greater than the diameter of the airway (air takes the path of least resistance).

2. How should the cervical spine of a trauma patient be protected during airway maneuvers?

The cervical spine of a trauma patient should not be allowed to move during airway management procedures. Manual in-line stabilization is superior to a cervical collar alone.

3. What are the options for airway management of conscious and unconscious trauma patients?

Suction should always be available for any trauma patient with the potential for airway compromise (immobilized patient, altered level of responsiveness). Conscious patients may tolerate a nasal pharyngeal airway. Unconscious patients may be temporarily managed with an oral pharyngeal airway and should be intubated when manual stabilization, personnel, and equipment are available. Intubation devices that do not require direct visualization may help limit neck movement.

4. After definitive airway management, what techniques should be used to confirm proper airway device placement?

Listening for presence of breath sounds in all four quadrants of the chest is the first and most rapid confirmation of proper airway adjunct placement. End-tidal carbon dioxide detection with either disposable or continuous monitoring device can provide evidence for pulmonary gas exchange. The esophageal tube detector returns air from a tracheally placed tube. The detector collapses the esophagus, preventing withdrawal of air from an esophageally placed tube. Chest x-ray will provide visual evidence of tube location. Oxygen saturation monitoring provides a remote measure of the effectiveness of ventilation.

CHEST TRAUMA

5. List the potential problems of blunt chest trauma from A to J.

A = Aortic transection or tear
B = Bronchial tear or rupture
C = Cord (spinal) injury
D = Diaphragmatic rupture
E = Esophageal injury
F = Flail chest or rib fracture
G = Gas in the chest or pneumothorax
H = Hemothorax
I = Infarction from myocardial contusion
J = Jugular venous distention from cardiac tamponade

6. What clues to chest injury can be obtained from observation of a damaged vehicle?

Damage to the interior of the vehicle may suggest damage to the body parts that contacted these surfaces. Steering wheel damage suggests flail chest, sternal fracture, pulmonary contusion, cardiac contusion, aortic tear, and tracheobronchial injury. Deformation of a door or post into the passenger compartment suggests damage to the lateral chest wall, rib fracture, pulmonary contusion, and pneumo- or hemothorax. Unrestrained objects within the passenger compartment may cause penetrating or blunt trauma.

7. At what anatomic level can penetrating trauma affect the chest, abdomen, or both?

The diaphragm is a dome-shaped organ. All injuries between the levels of T4 and L1 should be considered both chest and abdominal injuries until proved otherwise, with consideration of movement and position of the diaphragm at the time of injury. In the case of penetrating trauma, missiles may traverse the lung, diaphragm, abdominal contents, and retroperitoneal space before exiting the body.

8. What clues to chest injury can be obtained from observation of the appearance and movement of the anterior chest wall?

Clues include ecchymosis along the path of the seat belt, arc-shaped bruises across the chest from the steering wheel, steering column injuries to the sternum, and bruising along the inferior border of the ribs that may suggest liver and spleen injury. Careful observation of the chest wall may reveal asymmetrical movement. Lack of expansion of one side of the chest suggests tension pneumothorax. Severe tension pneumothorax may cause bulging of the intercostal spaces. Paradoxical movement or seesaw effect may reveal a flail segment. Accessory muscle use provides information about how much effort the patient must expend to move air.

9. What associated injuries should be anticipated when a rib fracture is present? What diagnostic procedures should be anticipated?

Injuries to the lung beneath the rib should be anticipated. If the lung surface is penetrated, air or blood may leak into the pleural space, causing a pneumo- or hemothorax. Pneumothorax, hemothorax, pulmonary contusion, and injuries to the liver and spleen are most common. However, cardiac contusion and injuries to great vessels also may occur and can be ruled out by initial chest x-ray, computed tomography (CT), or angiography.

10. What specific rib injuries are associated with a flail chest?

A flail chest occurs when each of three or more adjacent ribs is fractured in at least two places.

11. What observations suggest a flail chest?
- Paradoxical chest wall movement
- Dyspnea
- Hypoxia
- Cyanosis
- Chest wall pain
- Decreased oxygen saturation

12. What is the preferred method for initial treatment of a flail chest?

Initial management of the flail chest should include manual stabilization and splinting of the flail segment with a bulky dressing or rigid splint. The patient may be rolled on the affected side in the case of a posterior or lateral injury. Intubation and mechanical ventilation are often required.

13. What associated injuries should be anticipated with flail chest?

Injuries commonly associated with a flail chest include pneumo- or hemothorax and perhaps cardiac contusion if the sternum is involved. Pulmonary contusion is almost always present.

14. What factor helps to predict the risk of complications from the treatment of flail chest?

The duration of mechanical ventilatory support is correlated with the risk of complications and poor outcome.

15. What injuries may be suspected solely from observation of the chest wall?
- Uneven rise and fall of the chest wall during respiration may suggest pneumothorax, tension pneumothorax, or flail chest.
- Entrance and exit wounds can be discovered.
- Ecchymosis or abrasion may overlie rib injuries.
- A line of demarcation across the chest that demonstrates pink, dry skin below and gray, clammy skin above suggests a spinal cord injury somewhere in the thoracic spine.

16. What is the most common chest injury among the elderly?

Rib fractures are common in elderly patients because of the brittle nature of older bones and the loss of overlying soft tissue for protection.

17. What is the most common complication of rib fractures in elderly patients? How can it be prevented?

Rib fractures pose a particular problem in the elderly because of the high incidence of pneumonia related to inactivity and decreased tidal volume. Special attention should be paid to ensuring that a well-informed and responsible attendant accompanies the patient home or that the patient is admitted for observation for underlying injury. Frequent lung expansion (even though it hurts) by deep breathing or coughing can reduce the incidence of pneumonia. Some pain reduction strategies that may facilitate deep breathing and coughing include support pillows for manual splinting, positioning, and premedication.

18. Why is a rib fracture in a child more significant than a similar injury in an adult?

Because children's ribs are so elastic and resistant to fracture, a positive diagnosis should alert the trauma team that the child has suffered a significant forceful injury. The suspicion of underlying injuries should be very high.

19. What are the common causes of sternal fractures? What findings suggest their presence?

Cardiopulmonary resuscitation (CPR), impact with the steering wheel, and impact with the seat belt harness are the most common causes of sternal fracture. Localized pain, dyspnea, crepitus, and hypoventilation (due to pain) are usually seen.

20. What clues other than mechanism of injury and shock suggest a hemothorax?

Any patient with a penetrating chest injury should be considered to have hemothorax.

21. How can blood from a hemothorax be recycled for patient use?

Autotransfusion systems that include chest drainage units with a feature that allows the recovery of shed blood may be used to provide the patient's own blood for autotransfusion.

22. What factors related to fluid resuscitation should be considered in patients with a chest injury who are in shock?

As with all trauma patients, we must determine what is going to kill the patient first and make it the priority of care. Usually hypotension is the highest priority, but when the patient is aggressively resuscitated with large fluid volumes, careful monitoring must be conducted. Fluid administration rates must be decreased to a modest infusion when the patient is determined to be hemodynamically stable. If fluid resuscitation is overly aggressive, pulmonary edema may occur. Hypothermia is another possible complication of administration of large volumes of fluids; it can be avoided by using fluid-warming devices.

PULMONARY TRAUMA

23. What information can be gathered from listening to breath sounds?

Unequal breath sounds or absence of breath sounds in the presence of pneumothorax or hemothorax suggests that the lung is partially collapsed, that blood has accumulated in the pleural space, or that an airway adjunct was not placed properly.

24. What percentage of patients with chest injury can be managed without surgical intervention?

More than 85% of thoracic trauma can be managed with a chest tube to facilitate drainage of air or blood from the pleural space to reduce pneumo- or hemothorax.

25. How are accessory muscles used to assist ventilation?

Accessory muscles are used when the normal contraction of the diaphragm is insufficient to increase intrathoracic volume to move an adequate tidal volume. The intercostal muscles expand the chest wall diameter; the sternocleidomastoid muscles elevate the clavicle and first rib to increase intrathoracic volume.

26. What behavioral factors increase the risk of spontaneous pneumothorax?

- Marijuana use. "Bong lung" describes the spontaneous pneumothorax that develops when a person coughs or forcefully exhales against a closed glottis, resulting in high intrathoracic pressures that may rupture a bleb.
- Overexertion, particularly in an unfit person, may create the same phenomenon.
- Cigarette smokers and patients with chronic obstructive pulmonary disease are also prone to bleb formation, coughing, and rupture with pneumothorax development.

27. What can Timmy teach us about pulmonary contusions?

Timmy was a 17-year-old patient whose chest was run over by a dual-axle truck outfitted as a float in a parade. He suffered no rib fractures, but pulmonary contusion was so significant that he required a total of 17 chest tubes and 2½ months on a ventilator. Lesson? Adolescents and children have flexible ribs, and the absence of rib fractures does not rule out significant intrathoracic injury.

28. During the development of a tension pneumothorax, what is the common sequence of cardiovascular and respiratory changes?

The patient first experiences pain and mild shortness of breath, which progresses to severe dyspnea with extreme respiratory effort, notable decrease in breath sounds on the affected side, hypotension, hypoxia, distended jugular veins, and deviated trachea.

29. Describe the procedure for emergency treatment of tension pneumothorax using commercially available or improvised equipment.

Needle decompression of the chest can be a life-saving emergency intervention. Kits are available, or improvised devices can be made from a 14-gauge, 2-inch catheter placed over the needle IV device. A one-way valve can be made from a syringe barrel, glove finger, or Penrose drain. The chest wall is entered over the top of the third rib (second intercostal space) in the mid-clavicular line. Caution is necessary to avoid the inferior border of the rib above, where the intercostal artery and nerve are located. Nurses in the prehospital or rural environment may be the only providers present and can perform this life-saving procedure. Protocols should be prepared in advance to address scope of practice concerns.

30. What type of chest injury presents with the sound of air movement through the chest wall? Describe the nursing treatment of this injury. What observations should cause you to question the effectiveness of treatment? How should you respond?

An open or "sucking" chest wound describes the ability of air to enter the pleural space through an opening in the chest wall. The opening should be sealed with an occlusive dressing taped on three sides. Air should be able to move out of but not into the wound/dressing. Severe dyspnea, tachycardia, neck vein distention, decreased or absent breath sounds, or tracheal deviation may indicate that the dressing has become sealed to the chest wall, allowing a tension pneumothorax to develop. The dressing should be released to allow the escape of air.

31. What clinical findings suggest tracheobronchial injury?
Mediastinal "crunch" and pain, dyspnea, hypoxia, and mediastinal air visible on chest x-ray are signs of tracheobronchial injury.

32. What history or assessment findings suggest esophageal injury?
Suspect esophageal injury when the exam reveals subcutaneous emphysema in the neck, resulting in airway compromise due to crowding from esophageal edema. Also be concerned with impalement injuries through the mouth (e.g., when a child falls on a stick in the mouth) or penetrating injuries to the neck.

CARDIAC AND THORACIC VASCULAR TRAUMA

33. For patients with a clavicle or first rib fracture, what associated injuries and radiologic procedures may be anticipated?
The subclavian artery and vein lie beneath the clavicle and first rib and are frequently damaged. Chest x-ray may reveal a hemothorax, but arteriography is usually required to visualize the vascular structures. One should be suspicious of any bruising at the base of the neck, clavicular pain or deformity, or difficulty in moving the shoulder.

34. What two injuries commonly underlie sternal fracture?
Cardiac contusion and aortic injury are associated with a very high-speed deceleration mechanism that fractures the sternum.

35. What findings help to differentiate tension pneumothorax and pericardial tamponade?
Signs of tension pneumothorax and pericardial tamponade are often similar. In general, both result from a significant mechanism of injury, and both demonstrate acute shortness of breath and chest pain, hypoxia and profound hypotension, distended neck veins, and signs of inadequate organ perfusion. Improvement after needle thoracostomy or chest tube insertion suggests tension pneumothorax. Resistance when the intubated patient is ventilated indicates that the problem is most likely pulmonary in origin. Lack of improvement after needle thoracostomy or chest tube insertion, muffled heart tones, and blood in the pericardium when pericardiocentesis is done suggest cardiac tamponade.

36. What is Beck's triad in cardiac tamponade?
Beck's triad includes hypotension, muffled heart tones, and distended neck veins.

37. What other physical findings suggest cardiac tamponade?
Pericardial friction rub, precordial pain, and progressive tachycardia are early signs. Pulsus paradoxus may develop as constriction increases. Fever and leukocytosis may develop during hospitalization.

38. Define pulsus paradoxus. How is it assessed?
Pulsus paradoxus refers to a significant decrease in systolic blood pressure during inspiration. To make this assessment, the nurse should slowly deflate the blood pressure cuff at a rate of 2 mmHg per heartbeat. Note the pressure at the first Korotkoff sound (during expiration), and then note the pressure when these sounds are heard during both expiration and inhalation. If there is a difference of 10 mmHg or more, pulsus paradoxus is present. Pulsus paradoxus can indicate cardiac tamponade, great vessel compression, constrictive pericarditis, or severe emphysema.

39. What electrocardiographic (ECG) change is associated with cardiac tamponade?

Electrical alternans is a term used to describe the alternating QRS amplitude associated with cardiac tamponade. Low voltages are also common on the 12-lead ECG.

40. How should the nurse prepare for a pericardiocentesis? What is the nurse's role during the procedure? How can you determine whether the aspirated blood is from the pericardium or the heart?

1. Prepare an 18-gauge spinal needle on a 60-ml syringe, and attach a 3-way stopcock.
2. Connect the red ECG lead (lead II) to the needle with an alligator clip.
3. Observe the monitor for a current of injury (ST elevation or spike) indicating that the myocardium has been touched by the needle.
4. When the current of injury is noted, the physician should retreat the needle slightly while withdrawing the plunger on the syringe.
5. Blood from the pericardium can be removed until normal heart function is restored.

41. What is the mortality rate for cardiac tamponade?

The mortality rate for cardiac tamponade is 50%.

42. What ECG findings are associated with myocardial contusion?

ECG findings may be similar to those for myocardial infarction, including ST elevation or depression, flipped T waves, and Q waves. A normal ECG does not rule out myocardial contusion, just as a normal ECG does not rule out myocardial infarction.

43. Are cardiac enzymes useful in the diagnosis of myocardial contusion?

Troponin I and troponin T are cardiac-specific enzymes that are often elevated after myocardial contusion. Creatine kinase-MB is less specific and often elevated after chest trauma.

44. What blunt chest injury is almost always fatal?

Cardiac rupture is almost always fatal.

45. What assessment clues suggest an aortic tear or dissection?

Mechanism of injury; profound, rapidly progressing hypovolemic shock; and widened mediastinum or aortic shadow on chest x-ray may suggest aortic injury. The diagnosis is confirmed with arteriography.

DIAPHRAGMATIC TRAUMA

46. How does an understanding of the mechanics of respiration help to explain the body's response to chest trauma?

When the mechanism of the bellows is disrupted by injury, the lungs, which are completely dependent on the muscles of respiration for inflation and deflation, do not function normally. Any injury to the muscular or bony structure of the chest is likely to have an adverse effect on pulmonary function.

47. Why is diaphragmatic rupture potentially life-threatening? What common nursing intervention may help to reduce excessive chest pressure and improve ventilation?

Abdominal contents may be pushed through the rupture into the chest cavity, mechanically compressing the lungs and thus reducing tidal volume. A nasogastric tube can decompress the stomach, allowing lung reexpansion.

VENTILATOR MANAGEMENT

48. How do chronic lung conditions affect patients with chest injuries?

Patients with chronic lung disease have limited lung function and respiratory reserves, placing them at increased risk for the following complications:

- Respiratory failure
- Pneumothorax
- Acute respiratory distress syndrome (ARDS)
- Difficult ventilatory management

49. What are the standard ventilator settings that nurses can use as a frame of reference?

A set of common initial ventilator settings may look like the following:
- Mode: assist control
- Tidal volume: 10–12 ml/kg (e.g., 800 ml in a 70-kg patient)
- Rate: 16 breaths per minute
- Fractional concentration of oxygen in inspired gas (FIO_2): 100% initially; then adjusted based on blood gasses
- Positive end-expiratory pressure (PEEP): none (may be used starting at 2.5 cmH_2O for pulmonary edema and ARDS)

50. What should I do if the ventilator does not seem to be functioning properly and the patient is in distress?

The ventilator is a mechanical version of the bag-valve device. Simply disconnect the ventilator tubing and ventilate the patient with the bag-valve device. Call the respiratory therapist or other assistance to manage the ventilator while you help the patient breathe.

BIBLIOGRAPHY

1. McQuillan KA, et al (eds): Trauma Nursing: From Resuscitation through Rehabilitation, 3rd ed. Philadelphia, Mosby, 2002.
2. Naude GP, Bongard ES, Demetriades D (eds): Trauma Secrets. Philadelphia, Hanley & Belfus, 1999.
3. Neff JA, Kidd PS: Trauma Nursing. St. Louis, Mosby, 1993.

9. ABDOMINAL AND GENITOURINARY TRAUMA

Ruth Paiano, MS, ARNP

1. How does blunt trauma injure the abdomen?

The compression and deceleration of blunt trauma lead to fractures of solid organ capsules and parenchyma. The hollow organs can collapse and absorb more force.

2. Describe the general differences in injuries to solid vs. hollow organs.

In general, solid organs respond to trauma by bleeding. Hollow organs often rupture and release their contents into the peritoneal cavity, causing inflammation and infection.

3. What is the most common solid organ abdominal injury?

The liver.

4. What hollow abdominal organ is most commonly injured?

The small bowel.

5. What abdominal injuries commonly result from seat belts?

Small bowel and colon injuries result most frequently from a sudden increase in intraluminal pressure or shearing forces due to rapid deceleration. Liver, spleen, and pancreas injuries occur with less frequency.

6. What positive findings are important to document on the abdominal assessment of a trauma patient?

- Appearance (distention, ecchymoses, lap-belt signs, abrasions, lacerations, wounds)
- Auscultation (bowel sounds, bruits)
- Tenderness (guarding, rebound)
- Palpation (organomegaly, pulsating masses)

7. What is diagnostic peritoneal lavage (DPL)?

DPL is a quick procedure to diagnose intra-abdominal bleeding.

8. When should DPL, computed tomography (CT) scan, and focused abdominal sonography for trauma (FAST) be used for diagnosis?

TEST	INDICATIONS/ADVANTAGES	DISADVANTAGES
DPL	Triage hemodynamically unstable patients with multiple injuries in blunt and penetrating trauma Detect diaphragmatic injuries in penetrating trauma and depth of penetration in gunshot wounds	Complications: infection, hematoma, intraperitoneal perforation
CT	Stable trauma patients with blunt injury Patients with penetrating trauma and suspected retroperitoneal injury	Low sensitivity for diagnosing hollow viscus and diaphragmatic injury in penetrating trauma
FAST	Identify the presence of fluid in the abdomen Rapidly identify the peritoneal cavity as a source of significant hemorrhage for patients too unstable to go to CT Evaluate patients without major risk factors for abdominal injury who do not require more extensive evaluation	Does not image solid parenchymal damage, retroperitoneum, or diaphragmatic injuries well Poor recognition of bowel injury without hemorrhage

9. What is the nursing role in DPL?
- Insert a Foley catheter to decompress the bladder.
- Insert a nasogastric tube attached to gastric suction to decompress the stomach.
- Set up DPL solution, which should be warmed to prevent hypothermia.
- Assist with procedure.
- After the fluid is infused, place the solution below the level of the patient's body.
- Obtain samples.
- Monitor for complications.

10. What are the most common complications of DPL?
Perforated bladder, mesenteric vessels, small bowel and omental injury, peritonitis, and increased respiratory distress.

11. What are the normal values for DPL?

PARAMETER	RESULT	INDICATION
Aspirant	Gross blood > 20 ml	Positive
	Pink fluid	Intermediate*
	Clear fluid	Negative
Lavage fluid	Bloody	Positive
	Clear	Negative
Red blood cells	> 100,000 cells/mm	Positive
	50–100,000 cells/mm	Intermediate*
	< 50 cells/mm	Negative
White blood cells	500 cells/mm	Positive
	100–500 cells/mm	Intermediate*
	< 100 cells/mm	Negative
Amylase	> 175 U/100 ml	Positive
	75–175 U/100 ml	Intermediate*
	< 75 U/100 ml	Negative
Bacteria	Present	Positive
Fecal material	Present	Positive
Bile	Present	Positive
Food particles	Present	Positive

* Intermediate results require further patient observation and possibly repeat DPL based on patient's clinical condition.
Adapted from Bastnagel Mason PJ: Abdominal injuries. In Trauma Nursing: From Resuscitation Through Rehabilitation, 2nd ed. Philadelphia, W.B. Saunders, 1994.

12. In the multitrauma patient, what signs and symptoms should increase the suspicion of abdominal trauma?
Changes in the patient's level of consciousness from the scene to the emergency department may indicate head injury or intra-abdominal bleeding leading to shock. Any suggestive signs include patient complaints of lower chest, abdominal, or back pain at the scene.

13. When is exploratory laparotomy indicated in trauma patients?
In penetrating injury, physical signs suggestive of peritoneal injury; unexplained shock; loss of bowel sounds; evisceration of a viscus, including the omentum; and evidence of visceral injury, such as pneumoperitoneum or visceral displacement on x-ray.

14. What are the signs and symptoms of peritonitis?
Abdominal pain that increases with movement, abdominal rigidity, rebound tenderness and voluntary guarding, abdominal distention with diminished or absent bowel sounds, fever, chills, nausea, vomiting, anorexia, shallow, rapid respirations due to pain, and tachycardia.

15. What are the symptoms of an acute abdomen?
Distention, rigidity, and rebound tenderness.

LIVER INJURIES

16. What is the incidence of liver injuries due to trauma?
The liver is the most commonly injured organ in patients with blunt trauma. The incidence is estimated at 30–40%.

17. How are liver injuries stratified?

GRADE	INJURY	DESCRIPTION
I	Hematoma	Subcapsular, nonexpanding, < 10% surface area
	Laceration	Capsular tear, nonbleeding, < 1 cm parenchymal depth
II	Hematoma	Subcapsular, nonexpanding, 10–50% surface
		Intraparenchymal, nonexpanding, < 2 cm in diameter
	Laceration	Capsular tear, active bleeding; 1–3 cm parenchymal depth, < 10 cm in length
III	Hematoma	Subcapsular, > 50% surface area or expanding
		Ruptured subcapsular hematoma with active bleeding
		Intraparenchymal hematoma > 2 cm or expanding
	Laceration	> 3 cm parenchymal depth
IV	Hematoma	Ruptured intraparenchymal hematoma with active bleeding
	Laceration	Parenchymal disruption involving 25–50% of hepatic lobe
V	Laceration	Parenchymal disruption involving > 50% of hepatic lobe
	Vascular	Juxtahepatic venous injuries; retrohepatic vena cava/major hepatic veins
VI	Vascular	Hepatic avulsion

Developed by the Organ Injury Scaling (OIS) Committee of he American Association for the Surgery of Trauma (AAST). Adapted from Moore EE, Shackford SR, Pachter HL, et al: Organ injury scaling: Spleen, liver and kidney. J Trauma 29:1664, 1989.

18. How are liver injuries diagnosed?
Patients with gunshot wounds to the thorax below the nipple line require exploratory surgery. Patients with stab wounds below the nipple line who are hemodynamically unstable or who have abdominal tenderness also should undergo exploratory celiotomy.

In patients with unstable blunt trauma, DPL or abdominal ultrasound may be used to determine hemorrhage unless peritoneal signs require emergency surgery. In hemodynamically stable patients, CT scanning is often used to evaluate injury.

SPLENIC INJURIES

19. When should you suspect splenic injury in blunt trauma?
Splenic injury should be suspected with blows to the torso, especially to the left side. If lower rib fractures or left pneumothorax is sustained, the likelihood of splenic injury is high. Transient hypotension or decreasing hematocrit after injury indicates significant hemorrhage, and hemoperitoneum should be suspected.

20. What is Kehr's sign?
Kehr's sign is referred pain that radiates to the left shoulder or cervical region. It indicates diaphragmatic irritation and often can be elicited by placing the patient in the Trendelenburg position or palpating the left upper quadrant.

21. How are splenic injuries graded?

GRADE	INJURY	DESCRIPTION
I	Hematoma	Subcapsular, < 10% surface area
	Laceration	Capsular tear, < 1 cm parenchymal depth
II	Hematoma	Subcapsular, 10–50% surface area
		Intraparenchymal, < 5 cm in diameter
	Laceration	1–3 cm parenchymal depth without involvement of a trabecular vessel
III	Hematoma	Subcapsular, > 50% surface area or expanding
		Ruptured subcapsular or parenchymal hematoma
		Intraparenchymal hematoma
	Laceration	> 5 cm parenchymal depth or involving trabecular vessels
IV	Laceration	Involving segmental or hilar vessels and producing major devascularization (> 25% of the spleen)
V	Laceration	Shattered spleen
	Vascular	Hilar vessel injury with devascularized spleen

Developed by the Organ Injury Scaling (OIS) Committee of he American Association for the Surgery of Trauma (AAST). Adapted from Moore EE, Shackford SR, Pachter HL, et al: Organ injury scaling: Spleen, liver and kidney. J Trauma 29:1664, 1989.

22. What are the indications for splenectomy after trauma?
- Severe blood loss and hemodynamic instability
- With multiple injuries when time cannot be used for time-consuming repairs
- Irreparable injury to the spleen (grade IV and V injuries)
- Coagulopathy, hypothermia, and other conditions that prohibit prolonged surgery

23. What are the common complications of splenectomy?
Atelectasis, pancreatitis, postoperative hemorrhage, abscess formation, thromboembolic phenomena, and infection may occur immediately or several days to weeks after splenectomy.

24. What causes overwhelming postsplenectomy infection (OPSI)?
Encapsulated bacteria, such as *Streptococcus pneumoniae, Neisseria meningitidis,* and *Haemophilus influenzae* usually cause OPSI.

25. Who is at risk for OPSI?
The risk for OPSI is greatest in the first year after splenectomy but continues for rest of the patient's life. The risk is 2–10 times higher for children than for adults.

26. How can sepsis be prevented after splenectomy?
The Pneumovax 23 valent pneumococcal vaccine should be administered as soon as possible after a splenectomy.

27. What patient teaching is needed after splenectomy?
Patients need to know the signs and symptoms of infection and to understand the necessity of notifying their physician when these symptoms occur. Patients also should consider a medic-alert bracelet.

GASTRIC INJURIES

28. How common are traumatic gastric injuries?
The stomach is injured in approximately 20% of patients with penetrating intra-abdominal trauma. In blunt intra-abdominal trauma, approximately 1% of patients sustain stomach perforation.

29. What are the complications of gastric perforations?
- Generalized peritonitis followed by septicemia and disseminated sepsis if left untreated
- Subphrenic abscesses
- Leaking gastric suture lines
- Gastric fistulas

30. How can I tell whether fluid leaking through the wound or drainage site is due to a gastric fistula?
Test the fluid for pH. Fluid from a gastric fistula is acidic.

PANCREATIC INJURIES

31. When does clinical evidence of pancreatic trauma appear?
Clinical findings are minor in the first 2 hours after blunt pancreatic injury but usually progress and become significant by 6 hours.

32. If pancreatic injury is suspected, what should be monitored?
Serial assessments are necessary because patients with pancreatic injury develop significant epigastric pain radiating to the back, nausea, vomiting, and tenderness to deep palpation. Serial amylase levels also may be monitored for elevation over time to detect pancreatic injury.

33. What signs and symptoms are associated with duodenal or pancreatic trauma?
Acute abdomen, increased serum amylase levels, epigastric pain radiating to the back, and nausea and vomiting

34. Is serum amylase a reliable indicator of pancreatic injury?
Serum amylase may become elevated from parotid gland, pancreatic, duodenal, or genitourinary injury. Elevated serum amylase level is insensitive and nonspecific as a marker for major pancreatic injury.

35. How are pancreatic injuries graded?

GRADE	INJURY	DESCRIPTION
I	Hematoma	Minor contusion without duct injury
	Laceration	Superficial laceration without duct injury
II	Hematoma	Major contusion without duct injury or tissue loss
	Laceration	Major laceration without duct injury or tissue loss
III	Laceration	Distal transection or parenchymal injury with duct injury
IV	Laceration	Proximal transection or parenchymal injury involving ampulla of Vater
V	Laceration	Massive disruption of the pancreatic head

Developed by the Organ Injury Scaling (OIS) Committee of he American Association for the Surgery of Trauma (AAST). Adapted from Moore EE, Shackford SR, Pachter HL, et al: Organ injury scaling: Spleen, liver and kidney. J Trauma 29:1664, 1989.

36. List the most common complications of pancreatic trauma.
Upper abdominal abscess, pseudocyst, common duct obstruction, and peritonitis. Chronic pancreatitis may develop after multiple bouts of acute pancreatitis.

37. When should drains be removed after pancreatic repair?
Taking into account the mechanism and degree of injury, the drain should be left in place until the patient is eating, drainage is minimal, and the amylase level of the drainage is not greater than the serum amylase level.

DUODENAL INJURIES

38. How are duodenal injuries diagnosed?

The retroperitoneal location of the duodenum and pancreas make these injuries difficult to diagnose with DPL. A CT scan of the abdomen is a useful diagnostic tool.

39. What is important about the mechanism of injury in duodenal hematomas in children?

Duodenal hematomas in children are usually related to childhood play (falls or bicycle injuries) or child abuse. About 50% of duodenal hematomas are attributable to child abuse (i.e., the child is struck with fists or objects). Often medical attention is delayed until the child develops obvious signs of sepsis or hemodynamic instability. With a duodenal hematoma, bilious vomiting may be the only early clue.

40. Why is a profound inflammatory response associated with duodenal injuries?

Activated enzymes, bile, and the volume of fluid cause the inflammatory response. The alkalinity in the duodenum also produces immediate chemical irritation.

41. What complications are related to duodenal and pancreatic trauma?

- Peritonitis
- Pancreatitis
- Bleeding from a fistula eroding into vessels
- Systemic or intra-abdominal sepsis
- Pseudocyst
- Bowel obstruction
- Onset of diabetes mellitus (rare unless a total pancreatectomy is performed)

INTESTINAL INJURIES

42. What findings suggest bowel injuries?

Blood in the nasogastric aspirate or hematemesis may be the initial presentation for small bowel or gastric injury. Physical signs may initially be absent, and CT findings may be nonspecific. Diagnosis may not be made until peritonitis develops. Penetrating injuries usually cause a positive DPL. Subcutaneous emphysema over the abdomen indicates a ruptured bowel. In a recent study, not yet published, 50% of all patients with abdominal seat-belt markings had a positive laparotomy.

43. What are key areas of the postoperative management of patients with bowel trauma?

First assess and treat airway, breathing, and circulation (ABCs), then any concomitant injuries and complications. Key considerations with bowel injury include the following:

- Decompression and drainage of the bowel with nasogastric, gastrostomy, jejunostomy, or t-tubes
- Pain management (increased abdominal or referred pain may indicate infection, deterioration of an anastomosis, or ischemia)
- Maintain adequate fluid and electrolyte status. Bowel decompression may be necessary for an extended period. Close monitoring of intake and output as well as electrolytes is required to prevent dehydration and electrolyte depletion.
- Skin integrity can be impaired by drainage from the wound or fistula tracts. Maintaining patent drains and frequent wound assessment and dressing changes are helpful in maintaining skin integrity.

44. When are colostomies closed?

If all colon injuries are healed and the patient has no complications, the colostomy can be taken down in 1–2 weeks. Most colostomies are closed after at least 6 weeks of recovery.

45. Do rectal exams need to be performed on trauma patients?

The evaluation of rectal tone is an important part of determining the patient's neurological status and spinal cord injury. Other positive signs on rectal exams are gross blood (indicating hemorrhage), anterior tenderness (indicating peritoneal irritation), and palpation of a high-riding prostate (suggesting urethral injury).

46. How are rectal injuries treated?

Rectal injuries are often managed by fecal diversion with proximal colostomy and distal rectal washout. Once the injury is completely healed, the colostomy is taken down.

47. List postoperative complications associated with injuries to the stomach and small bowel.

- Peritonitis
- Postoperative bleeding
- Intolerance to tube feedings
- Hypovolemia caused by third spacing
- Fistula development or obstruction

ABDOMINAL COMPARTMENT SYNDROME

48. What is abdominal compartment syndrome (ACS)?

ACS is the adverse physiologic consequences of an acute increase in intra-abdominal pressure (IAP). Increased peripheral vascular resistance, decreased cardiac output, oliguria, anuria, increased airway pressure, decreased compliance, and hypoxia may occur. If ACS is left untreated, it leads to organ failure and death.

49. List the common causes of ACS.

- Blunt and penetrating abdominal trauma
- Accumulation of blood and blood clots in the abdomen
- Ruptured abdominal aortic aneurysm
- Hemorrhagic pancreatitis
- Pelvic fractures
- Hypothermic coagulopathy
- Septic shock
- Bowel edema from injury to mesenteric vessels or excessive crystalloid resuscitation
- Perihepatic or retroperitoneal packing for diffuse nonsurgical bleeding

50. What are the signs and symptoms of ACS?

The late signs of uncontrolled intra-abdominal hypertension (IAH) are the symptoms of ACS. Key components include elevated ventilatory pressures, elevated central venous pressure, decreased cardiac output, and tense abdominal distention. These components are reversed with abdominal decompression.

51. What interventions need to be initiated for patients at risk for ACS?

IAP can be measured via bladder pressures using a Foley catheter connected to a manometer system. This technique measures cmH_2O pressure. A pressure transducer provides readings in mmHg (1 mmHg = 1.36 cmH_2O). Normal IAP is close to zero. Hemodynamic status must be closely monitored. Moderately elevated IAP requires fluid resuscitation to restore hemodynamic stability.

52. How are IAP measurements graded? How do they correlate with clinical presentation and treatment?

See table on following page.

| GRADE | BLADDER (IAP) PRESSURE | | CORRELATIONS |
	mmHg	cmH$_2$O	
I	7–11	10–15	Significant alterations in physiology are evident, but decompression is rarely needed.
II	11–18	15–25	The need for treatment is based on the patient's clinical condition.
III	18–26	25–35	Signs and symptoms of ACS may develop insidiously, but patients usually require decompression.
IV	> 26	> 35	Signs and symptoms are overt, and patient requires decompression.

Adapted from Burch JM, Moore FA, Franciose R: The abdominal compartment syndrome. Surg Clin North Am 76:833–842, 1996.

53. List interventions for ACS.

For the nonsurgical patient, abdominal paracentesis may be required to reduce intra-abdominal hypertension (IAH). In surgical patients, primary closure of the abdominal fascia is avoided. The abdomen may be closed with a prosthetic mesh that can be opened or removed.

54. When can the abdomen be closed after decompression?

The abdomen is closed within 4–7 days after decompression. The patient should be hemodynamically stable after diuresis, with body weight near the premorbid level. If recurrent compression is likely, a staged closure may be performed with definitive closure at 3–6 months.

GENITOURINARY INJURIES

55. What injuries are most often associated with genitourinary (GU) trauma?

Pelvic fracture, lower rib fractures, gunshot wounds to the abdomen, and fracture of the transverse process of the lumbar spine are associated with GU trauma. Left kidney injury is associated with splenic injury.

56. What is a penile fracture?

A penile fracture occurs after a direct blow to the penis. The fracture is a traumatic rupture of the corpus cavernosum from the tunica albuginea. The patient presents with pain, swelling, discoloration, and deviation away from the lesion.

57. How is a penile fracture treated?

Conservative treatment includes urethral catheterization or suprapubic cystostomy, ice packs, elevation, and administration of anti-inflammatory drugs, sedatives, or analgesics. Surgical evacuation of hematomas and repair of the injury are other options.

58. What is the most common cause of a degloving injury to the penis?

Degloving injuries are often associated with industrial or farm machinery. The operator's pants legs get caught in the machine, engulfing the scrotum and/or penis.

59. How do you treat a zipper injury to the penis?

The treatment usually involves cutting off the zipper ends from the clothing and parting the zipper. Ice packs and analgesia should be considered for patient comfort.

60. What injury should be considered when a trauma patient has pain radiating to the testicle?

Pain referred to the testicle is compatible with a retroperitoneal injury and is seen most commonly with urogenital and duodenal injury.

61. What physical findings suggest urethral injury?

Blood at the urethral meatus, presence of a high-riding or absent prostate on rectal exam, and evidence of a perineal or penile hematoma are indicators of urethral injury. Passage of a urethral catheter is contraindicated if urethral injury is suspected.

62. What signs should increase the suspicion for bladder rupture?

Gross hematuria, inability to void, and severe tenderness in the hypogastrium in patients with lower abdominal trauma or a violent deceleration injury.

63. What is the most common concomitant injury with bladder trauma?

Pelvic fracture.

64. What organs and structures are located in the retroperitoneum?

Pancreas, kidneys, adrenal glands, ureters, aorta, vena cava, and parts of the duodenum and colon.

65. When a patient presents with a pelvic fracture, what other injuries should be anticipated?

Injuries to retroperitoneal structures, genitourinary structures, and pelvic organs or vessels.

66. What is the first indication of injury to the kidney?

Renal colic or costovertebral angle (CVA) pain. Severe CVA tenderness may be caused by ischemia from a renal artery thrombosis.

67. Identify the categories of acute renal failure (ARF)?

Decreased circulation and/or ischemia to the kidneys cause **prerenal failure**. Trauma patients are at great risk for prerenal failure with hypotension, hypovolemia, and cardiac failure.

Intrarenal failure includes physiologic events directly affecting kidney tissue structure and function. In trauma patients, nephrotoxic agents such as antibiotics or contrast media or rhabdomyolysis can cause intrarenal failure.

Postrenal failure includes obstruction in urine flow from the collection ducts in the kidney to the external urethral orifice or venous blood flow from the kidney. Primary trauma, such as ruptured bladder, disruption of ureteral or urethral integrity, or pressure from hematomas, causes postrenal failure. Other causes may include urinary retention from a urinary tract infection or neurogenic bladder.

68. List the stages of ARF.

STAGE	CHARACTERISTICS
Onset	An event initiates ARF. The kidney successfully compensates for changes in renal blood flow and filtration pressures.
Oliguric	Urine output is < 25–30 ml/hr with the presence of electrolyte abnormalities (lasts approximately 10–20 days).
Nonoliguric	Urine is poorly concentrated with a high output (up to 1 L/hr), electrolyte abnormalities are present, and creatinine clearance is low (lasts approximately 5–8 days)
Diuresis	Urine output is elevated (125–150 ml/hr), but the kidneys regain their function. Electrolyte imbalances are corrected, and urine is more concentrated.
Recovery	Restoration of renal function (requires 3–12 months, depending on the severity of the damage)

69. What are the negative consequences of improper pain management in patients with abdominal or GU trauma?

Trauma-related pain, primarily pain caused by thoracic and upper abdominal injury, causes decreased pulmonary function via chest splinting and reflex-activated diaphragmatic dysfunction. The consequent hypoventilation and atelectasis result in ventilation-perfusion mismatching and hypoxemia. Functional residual capacity, cough (i.e., forced expiratory volumes), and vital capacity are decreased with consequent retention of secretions, progressive atelectasis, and development of secondary pneumonia. Increased sympathetic tone from pain may decrease gastrointestinal tract motility, producing an ileus that complicates the delivery of nutritional support.

70. When a trauma patient's pain is managed with an opioid, what additional medication needs to be considered?

Opioids can cause constipation; a stool softener must be considered.

BIBLIOGRAPHY

1. Ferrada R, Birolini D: New concepts in the management of patients with penetrating abdominal wounds. Surg Clin North Am 79:1331–1356, 1999.
2. Hodgson NF, Stewart TC, Murray GJ: Open or closed peritoneal lavage for abdominal trauma? A meta-analysis. J Trauma 48:1091–1095, 2000.
3. Hudak CM, Gallo BM, Morton PG (eds): Critical Care Nursing: A Holistic Approach, 7th ed. Philadelphia, Lippincott-Raven, 1998.
4. Liolios A, Oropello JM, Benjamin E: Gastrointestinal complications in the intensive care unit. Clin Chest Med 20:329–343, 1999.
5. Marx JA: Genitourinary trauma. In Rosen P, Barkin RM (eds): Emergency Medicine: Concepts and Clinical Practice, 4th ed. St. Louis, Mosby. 1998, pp 555–582.
6. Mayberry JC: Bedside open abdominal surgery. Crit Care Clin 16:151–172, 2000.
7. McQuillan KA, et al (eds): Trauma Nursing: From Resuscitation Through Rehabilitation, 3rd ed. Philadelphia, Mosby, 2002.
8. Naude GP, Bongard FS, Demetriades D (eds): Trauma Secrets. Philadelphia, Hanley & Belfus, 1999.
9. Trunkey DD, Lewis FR (eds): Current Therapy in Trauma, 4th ed. St. Louis, Mosby, 1999.

10. MUSCULOSKELETAL TRAUMA

Sharon Saunderson Cohen, RN, MSN, CEN, CCRN

1. What three systems make up the musculoskeletal system?
1. Skeletal system (bones)
2. Articular system (joints)
3. Muscular system (muscles and connective tissue)

2. Assessment of a musculoskeletal injury should focus on what signs and symptoms?

PAIN	SENSATION	SWELLING	PULSE	ACTIVITY
Location	Normal	Location	Presence	Continued activity
Onset	Diminished	Amount/depth	Quality	Pain with activity
Intensity	Burning	Time occurred	Loss of (time)	Moves to command
Radiation	Tingling	Associated with ecchymosis	Diminished but palpable	Moves to pain/unable to bear weight
Quality	Numbness		With Doppler only	No weight-bearing

3. What is one of the most serious complications of a crush injury to extremity?
Compartment syndrome.

4. What is compartment syndrome?
It is an increase in compartmental pressures of an extremity that leads to compromised circulation and nerve function. The results of untreated compartment syndrome can be muscle necrosis, partial or complete nerve injury, and vascular compromise, which can lead to loss of extremity function.

5. What are the signs and symptoms of compartment syndrome?
Classic signs include pain, especially on passive flexion/extension of the foot; paralysis; paresthesia; and pallor. Some literature lists pulselessness as an additional sign, but pulses are present in most cases because the systolic blood pressure (BP) is much higher than the 30 mmHg needed to cause compartmental syndrome signs and symptoms.

6. What causes compartment syndrome?
Internal causes: fractures, vascular compromise (e.g., from a dislocation), reperfusion injury (e.g., crush or prolonged compression), any musculoskeletal injury, and burns.
External causes: constrictive dressings, including circumferential casts and splints. Military antishock trousers (MAST) and pneumatic antishock garments (PASGs) are rare causes. If the patient is ventilated, one of the first signs of compartment trauma may be increased difficulty in maintaining oxygen saturations.

7. What is the most common site of compartment syndrome?
The calf, followed by the thigh.

8. How is compartment syndrome treated?
Treatment includes fasciotomy, within 4 hours if possible. The procedure can be done at the bedside in an emergency or, preferably, in the operating room under aseptic conditions. Do *not* elevate the extremity before fasciotomy is performed; instead, place it at the level of the heart to promote arterial inflow.

9. Define Volkmann's contracture.

Undiagnosed compartment syndrome of the forearm may lead to contracture and paralysis. Richard Volkmann first documented this condition in 1881.

10. What is the best method to control bleeding?

Direct pressure is the best method to control bleeding. A tourniquet should be used as a life-saving measure only if bleeding cannot be controlled by other methods.

11. What is an avulsion?

An avulsion is full-thickness skin loss in which a segment of skin is torn away.

12. What are common mechanisms of avulsion injury?

Common mechanisms of injury include shear injuries (e.g., ejection from a motor vehicle) and industrial accidents involving heavy machinery.

13. How is an avulsion treated?

Because a large avulsion can lead to hypovolemic shock, always begin with the assessment and needed interventions for airway, breathing, and circulation (ABCs). In particular, monitor and control bleeding with direct pressure. Gentle irrigation of the flap is often necessary, followed by covering with a moist, sterile, bulky dressing. Definitive treatment may include simple closure, but a more extensive wound may require split-thickness skin graft.

14. Should you ever remove an impaled object?

No. More injury may result, especially large amounts of bleeding or nerve injury. However, an object impaled in the cheek often can be removed without sequelae.

15. Describe the treatment for an impaled object.

Depending on the location of the impalement, treatment may vary. Before definitive treatment, the impaled object should be stabilized, by whatever method works best, to prevent further injury.

16. How are fractures described?

Many terms are used, including descriptions of the following:
• Skin status (open vs. closed)
• Bone (proximal, medial, distal)
• Fracture pattern (e.g., spiral, comminuted)
• Degree of angulation or displacement (relation of the distal to the proximal aspects; e.g., lateral, medial, anterior, posterior).

17. What is the best method to immobilize a fractured extremity?

To truly immobilize a fracture, it is best to splint above and below the fracture, including the joints, proximally and distally. If definitive treatment is to be delayed, a well-padded splint is advised to avoid the potential for skin breakdown.

18. What should be assessed before and after splinting or casting?

At a minimum, assess CMS: circulation, motor, and sensory function distal to the fracture.

19. How is an assessment of extremity circulation performed?

Assessment should be performed distal to the injury. Circulatory assessment evaluates vascular integrity. Assess for capillary refill distal to the injury. If it is > 2 seconds, further evaluation is needed to find the cause and determine the appropriate intervention. Assess color of the tissue. Tissue should be pink, and skin temperature should be warm. Pulses should be noted for trends in quality and presence.

20. How is the neurologic status of an extremity assessed?

Motor and sensory assessments comprise the neurologic exam of the extremity. The nurse should assess for flexion and extension of the fingers or toes of the affected extremity and determine whether the patient can feel the fingers or toes. Gross sensation is documented, and further examination may be done, if warranted, to discriminate between one and two points and light and sharp touch.

21. What discharge instructions should be given to patients with crutches, cast, or any other orthopedic appliance?

The most important instruction is the need to assess neurologic and vascular status (CMS). Patients need to know whom to call or visit if a problem arises. If the patient is discharged with a cast, cast care instructions need to be given and documented. If the patient is going home with crutches, proper crutch walking (*not* running), including demonstration and patient performance, needs to be taught and noted. Any orthotic device (e.g., sling, sling and swath, splints) needs to be fully explained to the patient, including why it is needed, the proper fitting or use of the device, whether they can remove it to bathe, and how to reapply it.

22. What are the goals of fracture treatment?
- Alignment of the bones in both the angular and rotational planes
- Restoration of proper length
- Restoration of apposition of the bone ends
- Adequate immobilization
- Normalization of function

23. What treatments may the nurse anticipate for patients with a fracture?

Fracture treatment may vary depending on the location and degree of fracture as well as the age and premorbid condition of the patient. In general, five treatment methods are used:
1. No treatment or, at most, simple restriction of activity with a sling or crutches
2. Closed reduction followed by cast immobilization
3. Continuous traction, usually followed by cast immobilization
4. Open or closed reduction with internal fixation
5. Open reduction with external fixation

24. Describe the following patterns of fracture:

Angulated fracture: a fracture in which the two bone ends are at an angle to each other.

Avulsion fracture: a bone chip fracture caused when the tendon is pulled from the bone.

Buckle fracture: seen in children with bending of the cortex of the bone, but no disruption.

Closed fracture: intact skin over a fracture site.

Comminuted fracture: fragmentation of bone into more than two parts.

Displaced fracture: a fracture that involves *no* angulation—only displacement of the bone ends.

Greenstick fracture: seen in children; an incomplete fracture involving only one side of the cortex of the bone.

Impaction fracture: a fracture caused by compression forces at the site where the ends of the bone are driven into each other without fracture displacement.

Intra-articular fracture: a fracture involving the articular surface of the bone.

Oblique fracture: a fracture that creates an oblique angle to the long axis of the bone.

Open fracture: wound overlying fracture, through which the fractured bone (compound fracture) communicates with the external environment; high risk for infection.

Pathologic fracture: a fracture through abnormal bone (e.g., bone with tumor, osteoporotic bone, diseased bone).

Rotational fracture: a fracture in which one bone end rotates in relation to the other bone end along the longitudinal axis; most often seen on physical exam, not on radiographs.

Simple fracture: "clean break"; one fracture line dividing bone into two parts.

Spiral fracture: a severe fracture in which an oblique angle rotates along the long axis of the bone; caused by twisting.

Stress fracture: a fracture caused by repetitive forces unloaded onto the bone (as in competitive runners).

Transverse fracture: a fracture that is horizontal to the long axis of the bone.

25. What is the greatest risk once an open fracture has been identified?
Infection.

26. What initial treatment must be considered for an open fracture?
To minimize the infection risk, treatment consideration should include antibiotic therapy, tetanus prophylaxis, irrigation, and possible surgical debridement and stabilization of the fracture.

27. Define nursemaid elbow.
Nursemaid elbow is a radial head subluxation, usually caused by a pull of or fall on an outstretched arm. It occurs in children who have been pulled or swung by the arms.

28. What is tennis elbow?
Tendinitis of the lateral epicondyle of the humerus.

29. Define osteomyelitis.
Inflammation and infection of the bone marrow and bone. In adults, the most common pathogen is *Staphylococcus aureus*.

30. What is the growth plate?
The growth plate consists of the ends of the bone involved in bone growth.

31. Why is the growth plate of concern in pediatric fractures?
Injury to the growth plate of the immature or pediatric long bone may compromise normal bone growth.

32. Define the following terms of motion:
Abduction: movement away from the midline.
Adduction: movement toward the midline.
Eversion: sole of foot faces laterally or outward.
Extension: straightening of a joint.
Flexion: bending of a joint.
Foot dorsiflexion: foot upward at ankle, pointing to sky.
Inversion: sole of foot faces midline or inward.
Plantar flexion: foot downward at ankle, pointing to floor.
Pronation: palm down.
Supination: palm up.

33. What is fat embolism syndrome?
Entry of fat into the vascular system. The syndrome usually develops 24–48 hours after injury and most commonly occurs after a long bone injury.

34. What are the most common signs and symptoms of fat embolism syndrome?
- Change in level of consciousness
- Dyspnea
- High fever
- Petechial rash (usually over the thorax and upper extremities)

35. How is fat embolism syndrome treated?

Supportive treatment with operative stabilization of long bone fractures.

36. Why is a severe pelvic fracture potentially life-threatening?

High-energy forces that result in pelvic disruption also can cause associated injuries. With the pelvic injury itself, major blood loss can occur secondary to disruption of the large and numerous arterial and venous plexuses contained within the pelvis.

37. How is an unstable pelvic fracture stabilized?

There are several methods of pelvic stabilization. External fixation (e.g., with the Slatis or Pittsburgh frame or the C-clamp or "pelvic stabilizer") may be applied. The easiest method, but not always the most effective, is the use of MAST or PASG garments; when inflated over the pelvic region, they provide stabilization, especially in the prehospital venue. In addition, the astute nurse must treat for hypovolemic shock, initially with crystalloids, then with blood for large amounts of blood loss and persistent bleeding in light of pelvic bone stabilization. The newest device on the market for pelvic stabilization is the trauma pelvic orthotic device (T-POD).

38. What is the goal of pelvic stabilization in the emergent setting?

The goal of pelvic stabilization is to prevent the pelvis from further displacement and to control any bleeding by aligning the fractured bones to create a smaller space for blood to accumulate. This approach causes a tamponade effect to help control hemorrhage.

39. How many liters of blood can be lost in a severe pelvic fracture?

The retroperitoneal space (a potential space) can accommodate up to 4 liters of blood before tamponade can occur in adult patients. In an open pelvic fracture, there is no limit to the amount of blood that can be lost. Surgical hemostasis is imperative.

40. What type of anesthesia may be used for suturing a wound in the emergency department?

Local anesthesia or blocks are used for proper debridement, exploration, and closure of a wound. Local anesthesia (e.g., lidocaine with or without epinephrine), injected directly into the procedural area, is often used. If vasoconstriction is desired, lidocaine with epinephrine is injected. Bupivacaine (Marcaine) is an alternative anesthetic often used when longer duration of anesthesia is desirable. In addition, various blocks may be performed, depending on the degree of anesthesia required:

Field block: anesthetic is injected around the area to be worked on.

Digital block: used to anesthetize an entire finger or toe.

Regional block: used to anesthetize a larger area, such as an arm or below the waist.

41. Why should caution be used when anesthetizing with lidocaine with epinephrine?

Lidocaine with epinephrine has vasoconstrictive properties and should never be used (or very cautiously) on digits (especially distal), tip of the nose, penis, ears, or any other areas that are distal and thus susceptible to severe vasoconstriction that may lead to tissue ischemia and loss.

42. What are the differences in the various sutures used in wound closure?

SUTURE TYPE	SUTURE CHARACTERISTICS
Absorbable	Usually used for layers beneath the skin or mucosal surfaces
Chromic or plain	Absorbs quickly (7–10 days); tensile strength gone quickly
Synthetic	Causes less inflammatory response; tensile strength lasts longer
Nonabsorbable	Usually used for skin and subcutaneous pull-out sutures
Silk	Highly tissue-reactive; holds knots well
Monofilaments (nylon, propylene, steel wire)	Have prolonged tensile strength and low tissue reactions but require more ties to secure knot

43. What types of wound closure are used?

Primary wound closure is the immediate closure of a wound or laceration with sutures.

Delayed primary closure is suture wound closure usually 3–5 days after incision or injury.

Secondary wound closure is wound closure without sutures; the wound heals by contraction and epithelialization.

44. Is suturing the only form of primary wound closure?

No. Dermabond (Ethicon, Inc., a Johnson & Johnson Company) is a topical skin adhesive used for wound closure. Many types of skin-wound tapes (e.g., Steri-Strips, butterfly sutures) that approximate wound edges without actual suturing are also available.

45. What precautions should be taken in applying skin adhesives?

Skin adhesives are fast-setting and intended for topical application only. With use near the eyes, particular caution needs to be taken to avoid contact with the eye or eyelid. Do not apply liquid or ointment medications or other substances to the wound after closure with most skin adhesives because such substances can cause the adhesive to weaken; wound dehiscence may occur. For the same reason, do not apply skin adhesives to a wet wound.

46. What is replantation?

Replantation is the reattachment of a body part that has been partially or completely severed from the body.

47. Define warm ischemia time.

Time from loss of perfusion (usually time of amputation) to time of reperfusion (usually surgical replantation). Any period during which the amputated part is cooled down (placed in ice slurry) is *not* included. The longer the warm ischemia time, the less likely that replantation will be successful. Cooling the amputated part increases the potential for successful replantation.

48. Describe the emergency care of patients with a partial or complete amputation.

Emergency care of all patients begins with the stabilization and maintenance of the airway, cervical spine, breathing, and circulation (ACBCs). After stabilization of the ACBCs, care of the stump and amputated part includes the following steps:

Care of the stump or wound

1. Generously irrigate the stump or wound with sterile saline to remove gross contamination (no scrubbing or abrasive action). Do *not* use povidone-iodine (Betadine), hydrogen peroxide, or soaps.

2. Apply sterile gauze moistened with saline. If bleeding persists, apply a pressure dressing. Do *not* clamp or tie off any vessels.

3. Elevate the stump above level of the heart.

4. If the amputation is not complete, do steps 1 and 2 above, and apply a splint. Cool the devascularized portion of the affected extremity with ice packs. Do *not* let any tissue come in direct contact with ice. Elevate above the level of the heart.

Care of the amputated part

1. Generously irrigate the amputated part with sterile saline to remove gross contamination (no scrubbing or abrasive action). Do *not* use povidone-iodine, hydrogen peroxide, or soaps.

2. Place the amputated part in sterile gauze moistened with saline; then place in a clean, dry, airtight plastic bag or container. Place the container in an ice and water slurry (combination of both). Do *not* allow the amputated part to come in direct contact with ice. Do *not* use dry ice (which is too cold and freezes vessels) or salt.

BIBLIOGRAPHY

1. Aluisio FV, Christensen CP, Urbaniak JR: Orthopaedics, 2nd ed. Baltimore, Williams & Wilkins, 1998.
2. Brown DE, Neumann RD: Orthopedic Secrets, 2nd ed. Philadelphia, Hanley & Belfus, 1999.
3. Blackbourne LH: Surgical Recall, 2nd ed. Baltimore, Williams & Wilkins, 1998.
4. Emergency Nurses Association: Course in Advanced Trauma Nursing: A Conceptual Approach. Park Ridge, IL, Emergency Nurses Association, 1995.
5. Kitt S, Selfridge-Thomas J, Proehl JA, Kaiser J: Emergency Nursing: A Physiologic and Clinical Perspective. Philadelphia, W.B. Saunders, 1995.
6. Labus JB (ed): The Physician Assistant Surgical Handbook. St. Louis, Mosby, 1998.
7. Lopez-Viego MA (ed): The Parkland Trauma Handbook. St. Louis, Mosby, 1994.
8. Mercier LR: Practical Orthopedics, 4th ed. St. Louis, Mosby, 1995.
9. Naudé GP, Bongard FS, Demetriades D: Trauma Secrets. Philadelphia, Hanley & Belfus, 1999.
10. Sheehy SB: Emergency Nursing: Principles and Practice, 3rd ed. St. Louis, Mosby, 1992.
11. Skinner HB (ed): Current Diagnosis and Treatment in Orthopedics. Norwalk, CT, Appleton & Lange, 1995.

11. SKIN, WOUND, AND OSTOMY MANAGEMENT

Donna M. Matthews, RN, BSN, CWOCN

1. What basic components of wound care management does the trauma nurse need to know?

Crucial to wound care management are wound assessment, cleansing, closure (as appropriate), and discharge planning.

2. What are the outermost layers of skin called? What are some of their functions?

In assessing a wound, the trauma nurse must have knowledge of the anatomy and physiology of the skin. The **epidermis** is the outermost layer that generates cells, which promote wound healing. The epidermal appendages include nails, hair follicles, and sweat or sebaceous glands. The **dermis** is the next layer of skin and contains blood vessels, lymphatic vessels, nerves, and collagen. Both of these layers are vital to skin healing without the need for skin grafting.

3. What is collagen? Why is it important to wound healing?

Collagen is the major structural protein found in the dermis and is secreted by dermal fibroblasts. Collagen is important because it gives tensile strength, which makes skin resistant to tearing forces.

4. What layer of skin lies below the epidermal and dermal layers? What are its major functions?

The subcutaneous layer stores fat below the dermis and provides insulation against heat loss as well as protection from pressure and shear injuries.

5. Explain the three physiologic phases of skin or tissue wounds.

1. The **inflammatory phase** is a protective mechanism by which the body tries to repair itself. Inflammation is a nonspecific response to tissue damage caused by trauma or induced by other stimuli. It consists of a series of events, including vascular and cellular responses that begin immediately after injury and last for 3–5 days.

2. The **proliferative or fibroblastic phase** begins at 12–72 hours after injury. This phase includes collagen synthesis, angiogenesis, and epithelialization.

3. The **maturation phase** occurs 2–3 weeks after injury. New, stronger collagen is deposited in the wound.

6. What premorbid conditions may inhibit the physiologic response to trauma and put the patient at higher risk for infection and delayed wound healing?

- Acquired immunodeficiency syndrome (AIDS) or any immunocompromising disease
- Diabetes mellitus
- Leukemia and other cancers
- Steroids
- Chemotherapy
- Immunosuppressants
- Aspirin and nonsteroidal anti-inflammatory drugs (NSAIDs), which affect coagulation

7. What information should trauma nurses obtain about how a wound occurred?

The trauma nurse should ask the what, why, and when of injury. Of particular relevance are the mechanism of injury, time lapsed since injury, duration of any applied force (relevant to crush injuries), interventions before arrival at the hospital, past medical history, immunization status, and allergies.

8. What should be the primary treatment goals for the trauma patient with altered tissue integrity?

The primary goals are to preserve injured tissue, prevent or minimize systemic effects (hypovolemic shock), prevent infection, and identify and manage associated injuries.

9. In assessing the patient with soft tissue injuries, what associated injuries should the trauma nurse look for?

Any soft tissue injury increases the suspicion of underlying injury, such as a fracture, dislocation, or neurovascular compromise.

10. What types of acute wounds are seen frequently in trauma patients?

The trauma nurse often assesses and treats abrasions, abscesses, avulsions, lacerations, puncture wounds, and bites.

11. Describe the usual treatment plan for abrasions.

Abrasions (stage II wounds) are painful and exudative. The wounds should be gently cleansed with normal saline, and a nonadherent dressing such as Vaseline gauze should be applied to the wound bed and then secured with an absorptive gauze or Kerlix.

12. Give other examples of partial-thickness wounds (involving the epidermis and dermis) that a trauma nurse may assess.

In addition to abrasions, trauma patients frequently present with skin tears, carpet burns, floor burns, and road rash.

13. What are the necessary assessments and points of documentation in caring for a wound in trauma patients?

1. Size recorded in centimeters, including length, width, and depth. Also note any areas of undermining or tunneling, using the wound perimeter as the face of a clock (e.g., 2 cm at 4 o'clock).

2. The extent of tissue involvement, using the appropriate terminology. For example, partial-thickness wounds involve the epidermis and dermis. Full-thickness wounds involve deeper tissues. Pressure ulcers only are described as stages 1–4.

3. Anatomic location

4. Type of tissue in wound bed (i.e., necrotic or granulating)

5. Color of wound bed

6. Exudate, including amount and type

7. Condition of surrounding skin

8. Duration of wound

9. Picture of the wound with a ruler next to the wound for reference. Make sure that institutional policies for photography are followed.

14. What tissue compression injuries do trauma nurses frequently see?

Crush injuries, degloving injuries, and amputations.

15. What factors influence the severity of tissue injury from a compression mechanism?

The severity of damage is related to the type of tissue compressed, the length of time that force is applied, and the type of force applied to tissue.

16. What physiologic changes occur in tissues after a crush force injury?

The injured tissues undergo increased edema, third spacing of fluids, increased compartment pressures, and impaired tissue perfusion. The end result can be tissue ischemia and/or anoxia leading to tissue death.

17. What adjuvant wound therapy may be used for patients with crush injuries, compartment syndrome, and acute traumatic ischemia?

Hyperbaric oxygenation is the systemic administration of oxygen delivered under additional atmospheric pressure. It increases the oxygenation of tissue, as the amount of gas dissolved in a liquid is directly proportional to the partial pressure of the dissolved gas. Therefore, oxygen tensions can be raised 10–13 times higher than breathing oxygen at normal pressures. Hyperbaric oxygenation causes vasoconstriction and thus is useful in managing edema related to traumatic crush injuries. Although this concept appears to be contradictory by decreasing blood flow to an injured area, the increase in diffusion of oxygen overcomes the decrease in circulation caused by vasoconstriction, and wound healing is promoted.

18. What is a degloving injury? How should the trauma nurse care for it?

Degloving is a shearing force injury that results in the stripping of soft tissue from bone. It may be partial- or full-thickness loss and is mostly circumferential in tissue destruction. After pain control is achieved, the area should be irrigated with normal saline and kept moist with moist saline gauze.

19. What assessments of patients with a traumatic amputation are needed after stabilization of airway and cardiovascular status?

It is important to distinguish between a complete and incomplete amputation. Incomplete amputations exhibit some remaining tissue connection, whereas complete amputations are severed from the body. It is also important to find out whether the amputated body part accompanied the patient and whether it was properly preserved in ice to ensure early onset of cold ischemia time. (See page 100 for more information on amputation emergency care.)

20. What is replantation?

Replantation is the reattachment of a body part that has been partially or totally severed from the body. Examples include reattachment of bone, vessels, nerves, and tissue.

21. What role does ischemia time play in replantation of amputations?

Ischemia time is the period during which the affected part is not perfused. Warm ischemia time starts at the time of injury and ends when the amputated part is cooled. The longer the warm ischemia time, the less likely replantation will be successful. Six hours is usually the time limit. Cooled parts, however, may be replanted 10–12 hours after injury.

22. What factors are important to remember in considering the nutritional and immediate metabolic needs of trauma patients?

Patients with traumatic injury have an increased metabolic rate for 10–14 days after injury. The nutrient most in demand is protein.

23. What are the most clinically effective methods to cleanse a wound?

Wound cleansing is an area of controversy in wound management. Normal saline is an effective cleansing agent when delivered to the wound site with adequate pressures to ensure removal of bacteria. Pressures below 4 pounds per square inch (psi) are inadequate to remove bacteria. Pressures above 15 psi drive bacteria into tissue. One way to ensure an irrigation range between 5 and 15 psi is to use a 35-ml syringe with a 19-gauge needle or angiocath to irrigate the wound with normal saline.

24. Discuss the role of povidone-iodine solution (Betadine) and hydrogen peroxide in wound cleansing.

Many studies have documented that the use of antiseptics (Betadine, hydrogen peroxide, acetic acid) in open wounds is cytotoxic not only to bacteria but also to white blood cells and fibroblasts. Betadine is considered safe only as a preparation for intact skin. Hydrogen peroxide may be used when diluted with normal saline in a 1:1 concentration for initial wound cleansing of an area with an abundance of dried blood and other debris. Full-strength hydrogen peroxide is considered cytotoxic to wounded tissue.

25. Explain primary, secondary, and tertiary intentions in wound healing.
Wounds that are well approximated with little tissue defect and can be closed immediately are said to be closed by **primary intention**. Delayed primary closure is done 3–5 days after incision or injury. Wounds that are left open and allowed to heal by production of granulation tissue are said to heal by **secondary intention**. Wounds are described as healing by **tertiary intention** when there is a delay between injury and reapproximation of the wound edges.

26. What methods are used in primary wound closure?
Steri-Strips (wound tape) and topical skin adhesives (skin glue) are often used for facial wound closure. Sutures and staples are other methods used for primary wound closure.

27. What precautions should be taken when applying topical skin adhesives (skin glue) to a laceration?
Most topical skin adhesives are fast-setting and should be used with caution near mucosal tissue or near the eye (the nurse must avoid gluing the eyelid shut). Ointments or liquid medications should not be used on the wound after closure because they may dissolve the glue.

28. Do topical skin adhesives need to be removed like sutures and staples?
No. In most cases, by the time the glue wears off, the wound will be healed.

29. Is there any area of the body for which topical skin adhesive is not indicated?
Yes. It is not recommended for use over high stress areas such as joints.

30. A diabetic trauma patient recently received a large laceration to his lower extremity. What assessment findings may indicate serious wound infection? What are the likely causative pathogens?
A serious infection is present if the patient begins to complain of or show flu-like symptoms and has an extremely painful wound site with tense periwound skin that is swollen and shiny with purple, fluid-filled blisters. The infection is probably necrotizing fasciitis, caused by group A beta-hemolytic streptococci. Other causative organisms may include *Clostridium* and *Peptococcus* species, *Escherichia coli*, *Pseudomonas* species, *Staphylococcus aureus*, *Streptococcus pyogenes*, and *Serratia marcescens*.

31. What emergent treatment is needed for necrotizing fasciitis?
Treatment involves rapid administration of broad-spectrum antibiotics, surgical debridement, fluid resuscitation, and hemodynamic support if the patient is in progressive septic shock.

32. What key assessment findings should increase suspicion of necrotizing fasciitis (NF)?
The trauma nurse who can promptly recognize the possibility of NF can save lives by minimizing delays in treatment. Patients give a history of trauma, chronic leg ulcer, or a surgical incision. NF most commonly affects the extremities, abdominal wall, or perineum. The pain level far exceeds what is expected, and the wound is edematous. The skin is shiny, and the erythema spreads quickly. Subcutaneous crepitation and vesicles enlarging to foul smelling, exudative purple bullae should immediately alert the nurse to NF. Subcutaneous air is often visible on computed tomography (CT) scan, and lab work shows marked leukocytosis and elevated creatine phosphokinase levels as well as elevated liver enzymes and blood urea nitrogen. Even with optimal treatment, the mortality rate of NF is 40%.

33. Describe the treatment plan for patients with severe road rash.
Road rash is a large, painful abrasion. Pain control is essential before the wound is cleaned and sometimes even before the patient will allow assessment of the wound. Gentle removal of

road debris by using normal saline or a commercial wound cleanser containing surfactants is recommended. Unless the patient has an allergy to sulfa drugs, a silver sulfadiazine topical agent or similar preparation is applied to the wound and covered by dry sterile gauze or dressing.

34. When may a diverting colostomy be necessary in patients with abdominal trauma?

Injuries to the intestine from gunshot wounds, stab wounds, or blunt trauma may require a diverting colostomy to allow wound healing in the absence of fecal contamination.

35. In what type of bed should patients with acute spinal cord injury be placed to minimize the risk for acquired pressure wounds?

A bed with a firm surface that allows full spinal immobilization and performs continual lateralization.

36. In trauma patients with shock who are on vasopressive therapy, what must the intensive care nurse consider when using lower extremity compressive therapy for thromboembolism prophylaxis?

In all patients on vasopressor therapy, especially if the vasoactive drug causes peripheral vasoconstriction, the reperfusion time of the skin is extended. This principle applies to compression therapy in the sense that the period for which the compression device is left off the patient may need to be longer than in patients who are not on vasopressive therapy. If the skin does not get the needed time to reperfuse, skin breakdown will occur.

37. What is the best method of pin care?

Time has not solved this dilemma. Literature supports cleansing around the pin with various cleansers as well as no cleansing at all, with no consensus about the use of a cleanser or frequency of cleansing. There is some consensus, however, about the best method to avoid infection: let the pin "breathe." In other words, the tissue (or scab) surrounding the pin is moved slightly away so that the skin does not adhere to the pin. This approach allows any infection to surface rather than stagnate and tunnel inward toward the bone.

BIBLIOGRAPHY

1. Bryant RA: Acute and Chronic Wounds: Nursing Management, 2nd ed. St. Louis, Mosby, 2000.
2. Doughty DB: Principles of wound healing and wound management. In Bryant R (ed): Acute and Chronic Wounds: Nursing Management. St Louis, Mosby, 1992.
3. Hampton BG: Ostomies and Continent Diversions: Nursing Management. St Louis, Mosby , 1992.

12. SHOCK

Sharon Saunderson Cohen, RN, MSN, CEN, CCRN

1. Define shock.
Shock is inadequate tissue perfusion resulting in oxygen debt at the cellular level. Shock may be caused by failure of one of three components of the body that affect the delivery of oxygen and nutrients to the cells: the heart (pump), the vascular system (vessels), or the circulating blood volume. Ultimately, shock causes a decrease in cardiac output (CO).

2. Name the three types of shock.
1. Hypovolemic (hemorrhagic)
2. Cardiogenic
3. Distributive (also known as vasogenic).

3. What are the endpoints of resuscitation?
After frequent reevaluation of the shock patient, normalization of heart rate, blood pressure, and pulse pressure and improvement of mentation and tissue perfusion indicate stabilization of the patient. Because stabilization may not be permanent, continued evaluation and close monitoring are necessary.

4. How is CO calculated? What is the normal value? Why is it important?
CO = stroke volume (SV) × heart rate (HR)

The normal value of CO = 3 L/min in adults. CO serves as the primary compensatory mechanism for increasing oxygen delivery to the tissues when needed.

HYPOVOLEMIC (HEMORRHAGIC) SHOCK

5. Describe hypovolemic shock.
Hypovolemic shock results from acute blood loss or loss of plasma and extracellular fluids with the reduction of intravascular volume.

6. What are the most common causes of hypovolemic shock?
Causes of hypovolemic shock may include gastrointestinal bleeding, ruptured ectopic pregnancy, severe burns, or dehydration resulting from vomiting, diarrhea, profuse diaphoresis, or nasogastric suctioning. In trauma, it is the most common form of shock, resulting from acute blood loss (both overt and covert).

7. What is the most common sign of *early* hypovolemic shock?
An altered level of consciousness, particularly restlessness, agitation, or any central nervous system (CNS) depression. This simple but consistent sign in the awake patient is one of the earliest indicators of shock. Physical examination also may reveal nonspecific signs and symptoms such as cold, clammy skin, orthostatic hypotension, mild tachycardia, and vasoconstriction.

8. What are the common signs or symptoms of *late* hypovolemic shock?
Late signs of shock include change in mental status (e.g., coma), hypotension, and marked tachycardia. A word of caution: otherwise healthy adults with hemorrhagic hypovolemic shock, do not become hypotensive until as much as 30% of the blood volume is lost. Impending shock should be treated as quickly as possible, before the patient becomes hypotensive.

9. Why does tachycardia occur in hypovolemic shock?

Tachycardia occurs as a compensatory mechanism to maintain or increase CO and to improve perfusion to the vital organs and tissues. If SV decreases, HR increases to maintain CO. (Remember: CO = SV × HR)

10. Do all patients in hypovolemic shock experience tachycardia?

No. This question is tricky but important. Often elderly patients or patients with a known history of myocardial infarction are prescribed beta blockers, which block the compensatory mechanism of tachycardia. When an elderly trauma patient arrives in the emergency department (ED) with obvious blood loss, HR stays at 80 beats/min, and blood pressure (BP) is dropping, think of beta blockade. Even trickier is the patient who has a concomitant spinal cord injury and therefore cannot increase HR in response to blood loss and hypotension.

11. What is the best way to manage hypovolemic shock in trauma patients?

Warmed intravenous (IV) fluids and blood.

12. In traumatic hemorrhage, is it necessary to treat hypovolemic shock with IV fluids and blood?

Yes. But this therapy only buys time to get to the operating room (OR) for surgical correction of bleeding (which is the most probable cause of shock in trauma). The greater the patient's hemodynamic stability, the better the outcome. Controversial studies by Bickell et al. in 1994 showed that aggressive administration of IV fluids to hypotensive patients with penetrating injuries to the torso should be delayed until the time of operative intervention.

13. What is the preferred fluid for initial resuscitation of patients in hypovolemic shock?

Initially, an isotonic crystalloid such as lactated Ringer's (LR). Normal saline (NS) is an acceptable alternative, but prolonged administration may produce metabolic acidosis. Much controversy has surrounded the preferred fluid for resuscitation: crystalloids vs. colloids. Weinstein and Doerfler point out complications with crystalloid fluid resuscitation, whereas Schierhout et al. identify complications with colloid fluid resuscitation. Schierhout et al. conclude that neither fluid has shown superiority in any randomized trial; because crystalloids are considerably less expensive than colloids, use of crystalloids is recommended until further studies prove a positive difference.

14. In a trauma patient with hypovolemic shock, when is it best to start blood transfusions?

Studies of the exact timing for initiation of blood resuscitation report varying results. As a general rule, however, most trauma centers initially infuse 2–3 liters of LR, then begin blood if the patient remains symptomatic. These 2–3 liters of crystalloid infusion also allow time for typing and cross-matching so that the patient can receive type-specific blood.

15. If type-specific blood is not available, what is the blood type of choice to transfuse in an emergency?

Ultimately, type-specific blood is preferred, but when time is of the essence and the patient is in shock, the universal donor type O, Rh-negative is given. Often in male patients or women beyond child-bearing age, type O, Rh-positive blood is administered until type-specific blood is available.

16. What compound, found in circulating blood, is missing from crystalloid solutions or banked blood?

Banked blood (older than a few days) and crystalloids lack 2,3-diphosphoglyceric acid (2,3-DPG), which results in an increase in hemoglobin-oxygen affinity. As a result, the blood molecule will not easily release the oxygen molecule to the tissues.

17. What is shock index (SI) and how is it calculated?

$$SI = HR/systolic\ BP$$

SI may be a useful marker of acute critical illness. The normal value is 0.5–0.7. Values > 0.9 have been associated with injury or illness requiring immediate intervention.

18. Why would you assess orthostatic vital signs on a patient?

In addition to a complete physical examination, history, and baseline lab tests, assessment of orthostatic vital signs may provide clues that the patient has experienced or is at risk of experiencing a syncopal episode related to hypovolemia.

To test for orthostatic hypotension, obtain the pulse and BP after the patient has been supine for 5 minutes; have the patient then assume an upright standing position and note any symptoms of hypotension (e.g., dizziness, lightheadedness, feelings of near syncope). Standing measurements should be obtained immediately and repeated for at least 2 minutes. Orthostatic hypotension is generally defined as a decline of 20 mmHg or more in systolic pressure on assuming an upright standing position, along with clinical signs and symptoms. Some authorities state that a drop in diastolic BP > 10 mmHg, plus clinical symptoms, is a positive test.

19. What central venous catheter (CVP) value may indicate that a patient is in hypovolemic shock?

The CVP is determined by four components: blood volume, intrathoracic pressure, right ventricular (RV) function, and venomotor tone. Normal values are 6–12 cmH$_2$O. A CVP < 6 cmH$_2$O generally indicates hypovolemia. An elevated CVP, however, does not rule out hypovolemia. Certain pathologies, such as RV infarction or pulmonary embolism, can produce a high CVP, yet the patient has a low left-ventricular (LV) filling pressure and needs volume infusions. Like most numbers, the trend in the CVP readings with volume challenges is more helpful than absolute numbers.

20. How can the trauma nurse determine whether fluid resuscitation is adequate or more fluid is still needed?

Again, follow the CVP measurement trend. For example, if the CVP is low and volume challenge results in minimal change in the CVP, the patient is significantly hypovolemic and further aggressive crystalloid fluids are needed. If the CVP is normal, however, and volume challenge results in a rapid increase in the CVP with no improvement or a deterioration in hemodynamic status, the cause of the shock state is pump dysfunction and further volume infusion is not indicated. Fluid resuscitation, especially in very young, elderly, or renally impaired patients and patients with a poor cardiac pump, increases the risk for fluid overload. Reassessment of the patient is the key to successful fluid resuscitation.

21. Are military antishock shock trousers (MAST) indicated for control of hemorrhage?

In the trauma setting MAST garments do *not* improve survival; therefore, their use is controversial. Their application must not delay transport or fluid resuscitation. Currently recommended indications for use include splinting of pelvic and lower extremity fractures and control of associated hemorrhage and as a tamponade of intra-abdominal or lower extremity hemorrhage.

22. What is the most common form of shock in trauma patients?

Hypovolemic shock.

CARDIOGENIC SHOCK

23. Describe cardiogenic shock.

Cardiogenic shock results when the pump or heart becomes inefficient and can lead to inadequate tissue perfusion. The mortality rate is as high as 70–90% unless aggressive and highly technical care is rapidly initiated. Classic cardiogenic shock is related to systolic dysfunction or the inability of the heart to pump blood forward. This results in a decrease in SV and, therefore, a decrease in CO.

24. What are the most common causes of cardiogenic shock?

The heart can become inefficient for various reasons, including myocardial infarction (in particular, any significant loss of LV myocardium, especially in patients with ischemic heart disease), pericardial tamponade, and pulmonary embolus. Indirectly, a tension pneumothorax can cause pump failure and cardiogenic shock.

25. Describe the clinical symptoms of cardiogenic shock.

Symptoms vary with the cause of pump failure. Because of reduced CO, stimulation of the sympathetic nervous system, and decreased peripheral perfusion, nonspecific findings include cool and clammy skin, decreased pulse pressure with weak peripheral pulses, fatigue, weakness, and hypotension. Changes in level of conscious may include anxiousness, restlessness, and confusion. Pulmonary vascular congestion is frequently present and may manifest as dyspnea, labored respirations, rales (particularly in the bases), tachypnea, distended neck veins, and high CVP readings (> 15 cmH$_2$O). In more severe cases, frothy sputum or cyanosis may occur.

26. Do all patients in severe cardiogenic shock present with pulmonary congestion?

Your immediate answer may be yes, but after a bit of thought you should consider the possibility that the patient has suffered an RV infarction. Such patients may present in cardiogenic shock with clear lung fields.

27. What cardiac sound may be auscultated in patients with cardiogenic shock?

Typically auscultation of heart sounds is abnormal in patients in cardiogenic shock. A prominent S$_4$ indicates decreased ventricular compliance and, if accompanied by chest pain, suggests myocardial ischemia. An S$_3$ indicates increased ventricular diastolic pressure and congestive heart failure (CHF). In addition, a holosystolic murmur may be heard if mitral regurgitation is present. A systolic thrill and a holosystolic murmur, heard best at the lower left sternal boarder, are indicative of ventricular septal rupture.

28. What interventions may be expected in the resuscitation phase of patients presenting in cardiogenic shock?

Always begin with the ABCs (airway, breathing, and circulation). Allow the awake patient to sit upright to facilitate breathing, unless hypotension is severe. Consider endotracheal intubation if the airway is compromised or hemodynamic parameters are poor. If tension pneumothorax or pericardial tamponade is suspected, prepare for needle decompression of the lung or pericardial sac and placement of a chest tube in cases of tension pneumothorax. Attach a cardiac monitor, and immediately treat cardiac dysrhythmias that may contribute to the shock state according to advanced cardiac life support (ACLS) guidelines. Prepare for pharmacologic therapy to support hemodynamic function and maximize cardiac function. Additional medications may include dopamine and analgesia for chest pain. If pharmacologic therapy fails to support cardiac status, external or transvenous pacing may be necessary.

DISTRIBUTIVE (VASOGENIC) SHOCK

29. Describe distributive or vasogenic shock.

Distributive shock occurs when the blood vessels dilate. Distributive shock states include septic shock, neurogenic or spinal shock, and anaphylactic shock.

30. What causes distributive shock?

In **septic shock**, massive infection results in release of endotoxin that causes vasodilatation. In **anaphylactic shock**, a severe allergic reaction results in the following cascade: histamine release, increased capillary permeability, and dilation of arterioles and venules. **Neurogenic or spinal shock** occurs after a spinal cord or severe brain injury that results in loss or disruption of sympathetic tone and dilation of arterioles and venules.

31. With so many causes of distributive shock, are all clinical presentations the same?

Some symptoms are similar, but others are vastly different. The typical clinical presentations for the various causes of distributive shock are outlined below.

SHOCK STATE	HEART RATE	BLOOD PRESSURE	SPECIFIC FINDINGS
Septic shock	Increased	Decreased	With or without elevated temperature
Anaphylactic shock	Increased	Decreased	Respiratory difficulty
Neurogenic or spinal shock	Decreased	Decreased	Plegia from spinal cord injury or injury to medulla

32. What is the difference between high- and low-output stages in septic shock?

High-output stage refers to increased CO and decreased systemic vascular resistance, resulting in a hyperdynamic state (or early shock). Conversely, the **low-output stage** (or late shock) is a hypodynamic state in which CO is decreased and systemic vascular resistance is increased. Whether patients can be divided into one of these two groups is a controversial issue; it is more appropriate to view these processes as a continuum rather than distinct stages.

33. Do all patients presenting with septic shock have an elevated temperature?

No. Temperature elevation or hypothermia may be present in patients with septic shock. In neonates, immunosuppressed patients, or elderly patients, a subnormal temperature reading is often noted.

34. Describe the usual treatment of anaphylactic shock.

Definitive therapy for anaphylactic shock is directed at identification and removal of the antigen causing the allergic reaction. If a blood transfusion is the causative factor, the transfusion should be stopped. If the causative factor is exposure to a chemical or substance, removal of the chemical or substance is necessary. Treatment of the symptoms includes maintenance of a patent airway, effective breathing, and circulation. High-flow oxygen and IV administration of epinephrine, 0.1–0.5 ml of 1: 10,000 solution, repeated every 5–15 minutes, are used for profound vasoconstriction. Antihistamines (e.g., diphenhydramine [Benadryl], cimetidine [Tagamet]) or bronchodilators (e.g., albuterol, aminophylline) may be necessary in addition to IV fluids.

35. What is poikilothermia?

Patients with spinal cord injury (SCI) may have unopposed parasympathetic stimulation below the level of the SCI. This unopposed stimulation (no sympathetic opposition) often fails to maintain normal body temperature, allowing the patient to assume ambient temperatures.

36. Is the treatment for neurogenic shock similar to treatment for hypovolemic shock?

Unlike hypovolemic shock, which is a volume problem, neurogenic shock is a problem of arteriole and venous dilation. The volume is available but must flow through highly dilated vasculature, which results in venous and arterial pooling. Treatment begins with spinal cord stabilization concomitantly with the ABCs. Specific treatment may include fluids, but intravenous vasopressors often are needed to help constrict the vasculature and increase BP. As with any SCI, high-dose methylprednisolone is given intravenously within the first 8 hours after injury.

37. What physical signs often are seen as an emotional response to trauma?

Both patients and family members can experience a range of emotional responses to trauma, including anxiety, helplessness, depression, withdrawal, increased frustration, self-destructive behavior, and all of the physiologic findings connected with these emotions.

38. What ethical dilemmas arise from exsanguinating trauma patients who also are Jehovah's Witnesses and refuse blood transfusions?

The heaviest ethical dilemma is patient autonomy, which gives patients the right to choose actions that are consistent with their goals, values, and life plans, even if their choices disagree with the physician's. Most Jehovah's Witnesses carry pocket cards stating their beliefs or arrive sufficiently alert to express their views.

BIBLIOGRAPHY

1. Russell S: Hypovolemic shock: Is your patient at risk? Nursing April:34–40, 1994.
2. Blackbourne LH: Surgical Recall, 2nd ed. Baltimore, Williams & Wilkins, 1998.
3. Naude GP, Bongard FS, Demetriades D: Trauma Secrets. Philadelphia, Hanley & Belfus, 1999.
4. Lopez-Viego MA (ed): The Parkland Trauma Handbook. St. Louis, Mosby, 1994.
5. Kitt S, Selfridge-Thomas J, Proehl JA, Kaiser J: Emergency Nursing: A Physiologic and Clinical Perspective. Philadelphia, W.B. Saunders, 1995.
6. Emergency Nurses Association: Course in Advanced Trauma Nursing: A Conceptual Approach. Park Ridge, IL, Emergency Nurses Association,1995.
7. Sheehy SB: Emergency Nursing Principles and Practice, 4th ed. St. Louis, Mosby, 1998.
8. Goldman L, Braunwald E: Primary Cardiology. Philadelphia, W.B. Saunders, 1998.
9. Bickell WH, Wall MJ, Pepe PE, et al: Immediate versus delayed fluid resuscitation for hypotensive patients with penetrating torso injuries. N Engl J Med 331:1105–1109, 1994.
10. Schierhout G, Roberts I: Fluid resuscitation with colloid or crystalloid solutions in critically ill patients: A systematic review of randomized trials. Br Med J 316:961–964. 1998.
11. Schierhout G, Roberts I, Alderson P, Bunn F: Colloids versus crystalloids for fluid resuscitation in critically ill patients. The Cochrane Database of Systematic Reviews, Vol. 3. 1999.
12. Weinstein PD, Doerfler ME: Systemic complications of fluid resuscitation. Crit Care Clin 8:439–448, 1998.

IV. Special Populations

13. BURN TRAUMA

Kristopher G. Pidgeon, RN, MSN, CEN, and
Sharon Saunderson Cohen, RN, MSN, CEN, CCRN

1. What is the incidence of burn trauma in the United States?

Burn trauma is the third leading cause of injury death, and the U.S. has the highest incidence of serious burn injury of all industrialized countries. In addition, 10,000 burn victims die each year, and over 100,000 require prolonged hospital care or rehabilitation. The cost to society of the long-term morbidity from loss of physical function or associated psychological and cosmetic impairment is incalculable.

2. What are the causes of burn trauma?

Thermal (heat source)
Chemical
Electrical
Radiation

3. What organ is most affected by burn trauma? Why is this so significant?

The largest organ of the body is the skin, which is most affected by burn trauma. Skin is important to the body because of its diversified functions, all of which are vital to life. It is the first line of defense from infection and injury; regulates and maintains body temperature; prevents the loss of body fluids; and aids in the sensory interaction with the surrounding environment.

4. Define eschar.

Eschar is skin that has been made nonviable by burn trauma. It is also inelastic and can be quite restrictive. It is important to monitor areas of eschar because they may lead to neurovascular compromise of an extremity or restriction of the chest. If the chest is involved, impaired ventilation may result. Early excision or cuts to the eschar (escharotomy) are important to prevent compromise in the neurovascular status or normal chest expansion needed for adequate ventilation.

5. What is the priority of burn trauma resuscitation?

As with all trauma, the priority is based on systematic assessment and intervention for life-threatening injuries. Priority begins with the assessment of the ACBCDs: **a**irway with **c**ervical spine, **b**reathing, **c**irculation, and **d**isability (neurologic). Once the ACBCDs are stabilized, the priority becomes secondary assessment, which can focus on the extent of burn and the required amount of fluid resuscitation. The secondary assessment also should identify any and all associated injuries.

6. What type of shock is the most common after extensive burn trauma?

Hypovolemic shock is the most common type; it is caused by fluid and plasma shifts from the intravascular to the interstitial spaces.

7. Describe the pathophysiology of burn trauma.

After burn trauma the capillaries are damaged and become "leaky." Large amounts of fluids, electrolytes, and plasma shift from the intravascular space to the interstitial spaces. A burn that affects 15–20% or more of total body surface area (TBSA) causes hypovolemic shock if the patient is not adequately resuscitated.

8. How are burns classified?
Burns are classified according to the depth as follows:

BURN DEPTH	CLASSIFICATION	SIGNS AND SYMPTOMS	COMMENTS
First degree	Superficial partial thickness	Pain, dry, erythema, no blisters; involves epidermal layer only	Heals within 1–2 weeks
Second degree	Deep partial	Painful blisters, erythema, appears moist; involves epidermal and part of the dermal layer of skin	Healing from epithelization; often leaving blisters intact will prevent severe infection
Third degree	Full thickness	Dry appearance, dark, charred eschar, insensitive; involves all layers of the skin and some subcutaneous layers; insensate to touch but can involve severe, dull, pressure-like pain	Susceptible to infection; healing via contracture or skin grafting
Fourth degree	Full thickness	Involves muscle to bone; insensate to touch but can involve severe, dull, pressure-like pain	Amputation or major reconstruction is required

9. What determines the extent of a burn wound?
- The time in contact with the burning agent
- The temperature of the thermal agent (hot or cold) *or*
- The concentration of the chemical or radiating agent

10. What methods may be used to calculate the extent of the burn wound?
The extent of the burn wound is expressed in total percent of burned surface area (%TBSA) and depth. There are several methods to calculate the TBSA. The most common method used by both prehospital personnel and emergency departments is the "rule of nines." The body is divided into areas of 9%. Be sure to use the proper body map that corresponds to the age of the burned victim (see figure on following page). Another method is the palm of the hand, which is approximately 1%. A more precise and time-consuming method is the Lund-Browder chart (see figure on following page).

11. In the U.S. what is the most common formula to calculate the amount of fluid needed for resuscitation?
Aggressive fluid resuscitation techniques were not used until the 1960s and 1970s. The most common formula to calculate the amount of fluid needed to resuscitate is the Parkland formula:

Adults: 2–4 ml of lactated Ringer's solution × weight in kg × %TBSA injury

Children: 3–4 ml of lactated Ringer's solution × weight in kg × %TBSA injury

Give one-half of the calculated volume in the first 8 hours after burn injury (time starts when patient was burned, not when the patient received the intravenous line) and the second half in the following 16 hours. In addition to the Parkland formula, children need additional maintenance fluids that contain dextrose.

Like most formulas, the Parkland formula is to be used as a guideline to burn shock resuscitation. Additional parameters to ensure adequate fluid volume resuscitation include urine output, level of consciousness, vital signs, arterial pH, and hemodynamic parameters such as central venous pressure (CVP) or oxygen delivery (DO_2).

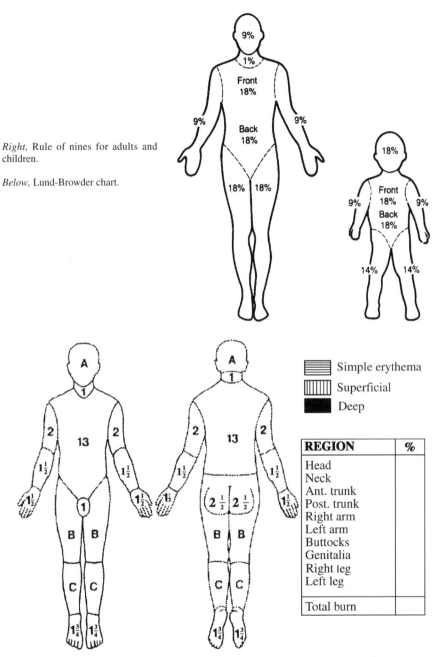

Right, Rule of nines for adults and children.

Below, Lund-Browder chart.

Simple erythema
Superficial
Deep

REGION	%
Head	
Neck	
Ant. trunk	
Post. trunk	
Right arm	
Left arm	
Buttocks	
Genitalia	
Right leg	
Left leg	
Total burn	

Relative Percentage of Body Surface Area Affected by Growth

AREA	AGE 0	1	5	10	15	ADULT
A = ¹/₂ of head	9 ¹/₂	8 ¹/₄	6 ¹/₂	5 ¹/₂	4 ¹/₂	3¹/₂
B = ¹/₂ of one thigh	2 ¹/₂	3 ¹/₄	4	4 ¹/₂	4 ³/₄	4³/₄
C = ¹/₂ of one leg	2 ¹/₂	2 ¹/₂	2 ³/₄	3	3¹/₄	3¹/₂

12. In the United Kingdom (UK) what is the more common formula to calculate fluid replacement?

Most UK burn units re-examine and recalculate the burn percentage using the Lund-Browder chart. Once the %TBSA is calculated, the Muir and Barclay formula is used to calculate fluid replacement:

$$\%TBSA \times body\ weight\ in\ kg \times 2$$

Fluid is replaced over the first 36 hours, which is divided into six periods because more fluid is lost from the body initially; leakage from raw areas slows down and edema is reabsorbed toward the end of the 36 hours. The period for fluid resuscitation is calculated from the time when the victim was burned, *not* the time when the intravenous catheter was started. At the end of each period, blood samples need to be taken to assess hematocrit (Hct) and to calculate the plasma deficit:

$$Plasma\ deficit = blood\ volume - (blood\ volume \times normal\ Hct)$$

This amount should be added to or subtracted from the calculated figure from the Muir and Barclay formula for the next period. The plasma deficit is then recalculated at the end of each period. Usually, a second crystalloid solution is started at a fixed rate to meet the patient's metabolic requirements during the 36 hours of resuscitation.

Like most formulas, the Muir and Barclay formula should be used as a guideline to burn shock resuscitation. Additional parameters to ensure adequate fluid volume resuscitation include urine output, level of consciousness, vital signs, arterial pH, and hemodynamic parameters such as central venous pressure (CVP) or oxygen delivery (DO_2).

13. Do all burn patients require fluid resuscitation?

No. Patients with burns affecting < 15–20% TBSA usually do not need fluid resuscitation. In the presence of concomitant bleeding due to trauma, however, the usual blood and fluid replacement is warranted.

14. Is urine output a reliable indicator of adequate fluid resuscitation?

In burns < 30% TBSA, a urine output of 1 ml/kg/hr may be a reliable indicator of adequate fluid resuscitation. In addition, the color may be indicative of the adequacy of resuscitation. Dark, tea-colored urine may indicate large amounts of myoglobin in the urine and thus inadequate fluid resuscitation. However, in larger burns (> 30% TBSA) urine output is not a reliable indicator, especially in the first 10–14 days. In the acute postburn period, urine output must be coupled with specific gravity and osmolality. In the addition to burns in a multitrauma patient, blood in the urine may be indicative of a pelvic or genitourinary structural injury. In the very old or cardiac patients or patients with larger burns, a pulmonary artery (PA) catheter may be indicated to monitor fluid resuscitation closely.

15. What are the advantages of a PA catheter placement?

A PA catheter allows improved guidance of fluid and blood resuscitation. It allows close monitoring of cardiac index, DO_2, and the patient's response to volume replacement.

16. After burn trauma the metabolism of the patient increases. How long does this response last?

Burn patients exhibit a hypermetabolic state as quickly as 1 hour post burn, and this response may last for several weeks. During this hypermetabolic state, massive protein catabolism and lipolysis occur. Meeting the metabolic demands can be a challenge, but it is crucial to optimize patient outcome.

17. What is the best route to meet the metabolic demands of patients with burn trauma?

Enteral nutrition is the preferred route and should be initiated after adequate fluid resuscitation. Maximization of both fluid replacement and nutrition reduces septic complication rates and improves survival rates. Enteral feedings should begin as soon as possible by placing a naso- or orogastric or small bowel feeding tube. Nutritional therapy should include nitrogen, omega-3 and omega-6 fatty acids, glutamine, and fiber. Feeding the gut prevents translocation of gut bacteria and fewer septic complications.

18. Discuss the role of antibiotics in the early phases after burn trauma.

Prophylactic intravenous antibiotics are not warranted because they serve only to select out resistant bacteria. Topical antibiotics should be used in second-degree (partial-thickness) and third-degree (full-thickness) burns. The most common topical antibiotic used in the U.S. is silver sulfadiazine (Silvadene). Silvadene has excellent coverage but may cause transient leukopenia.

19. Is elevation in core temperature a clinical indicator of systemic infection in patients with burn trauma?

No. Identification of systemic infection in most patients is based on the presence of fever, leukocytosis, erythema, and a hyperdynamic state. However, these signs are commonly present in burn patients in the absence of infection. Temperature elevations to 39°C are common. Hypothermia or a change in the established temperature pattern is a better indication of infection than simple temperature elevation. In addition, tachypnea and tachycardia result from metabolic demands of the trauma. The best indicators of early sepsis in burned patients are changes in established patterns. The patient who has an unexplained change in level of consciousness, new glucose intolerance, and recent onset of a new ileus is septic until proved otherwise.

20. What should the trauma nurse do if leukopenia develops in a patient using silver sulfadiazine?

Silver sulfadiazine has minimal toxicity, but it is a sulfonamide and should never be used in patients who report hypersensitivity to sulfa drugs. Minor skin rashes at the wound margins are common but rarely require a change in therapy. Significant leukopenia occurs in 10–15% of patients, usually 2–5 days after initiating therapy. Neutrophil counts < 1000/mm^3 are common but not associated with an increase in infection. Stopping drug application should stop the progression of leukopenia and begin the reversal.

21. Once the ACBCDs have been stabilized and fluid resuscitation begun, how does the trauma nurse care for the burn wounds?

If the burns involve < 10% TBSA, wet dressings can be used initially to help stop the burning process and provide some pain relief. If the burns exceed 10% TBSA, all burn wounds should be covered with a clean, dry sheet. Covering the patient with blankets may be necessary to avoid hypothermia. Applications of wet, cold, or ice onto large burn wounds may extend the depth of the burn and also induce hypothermia.

22. What are the signs and symptoms of inhalation injury?

Prehospital report, patient history, and a high level of suspicion are necessary elements in diagnosing inhalation injury. Other signs and symptoms may include one or all of the following:

METHOD OF ASSESSMENT	FINDINGS	COMMENTS
Visual assessment	Singed nasal and hair Carbonaceous sputum Burns in or around the mouth or nose Erythematous oropharynx, drooling with difficulty in swallowing	Suspicion should be higher if patient was burned in an enclosed space.
Auditory assessment	Stridor, hoarse, raspy voice	Usually indicates later finding of a partially occluded airway from edema. Prophylactic endotracheal intubation may be necessary to prevent loss of airway.

Table continued on following page

METHOD OF ASSESSMENT	FINDINGS	COMMENTS
Laryngoscopy	Supraglottic edema or erythema	Early prophylactic endotracheal intubation should be performed to prevent loss of airway.
Laboratory values	$\uparrow$ Carbon monoxide (CO) level $\downarrow$ Oxygen (O_2) level $\uparrow$ Carbon dioxide (CO_2) level	Although pulse oximetry (SpO_2) may show 100% on high-flow O_2, CO has 300 times greater affinity for hemoglobin than O_2. Treatment involves 100% O_2.

23. What is the ultimate challenge for the trauma nurse in caring for patients with burn trauma and inhalation injury?

Inhalation injury causes upper airway injury and has the potential to cause lower airway injury. Thermal injury results from direct heat exposure and is usually limited to the upper airway. Carbon monoxide (CO), a byproduct of organic combustion, is commonly inhaled. Since CO has a 300 times greater affinity for hemoglobin than oxygen, hypoxia may ensue. If hypoxia is left untreated, encephalopathy and renal failure usually develop. In addition, if chemicals and smoke are inhaled deep into the lungs, damage to type 2 pneumocytes leads to loss of surfactant production and alveolar volume. Coupled with this response is lung parenchymal injury that may result in "wet lungs."

24. Discuss the nursing treatment for patients with burn injury due to tar or asphalt.

Do *not* peel off the tar or asphalt until you have cooled it with cold water. Once the substance is cooled, the adherent tar or asphalt should be covered with a petroleum-based dressing to help dissolve the substance. Baby oil and mineral oil are cheap petroleum-based ointments that usually work well; mayonnaise works well also. Once the substance becomes soft, removal is relatively easy and priority can then focus on treatment of the burn wound.

25. What is the best approach to pain management in patients with burn trauma?

Pain management in patients with burn trauma is often unsatisfactory because of misconceptions about the sources of pain and optimal use of various analgesic agents. Quantification of pain severity depends on the patient's own assessment, using reliable and valid assessment tools. In addition, the presence of pain usually can be recognized from physical signs such as pupillary dilation, sweating, tachycardia, tachypnea, and increased blood pressure. The three general categories of management are early, late, and breakthrough pain.

26. How is early pain managed?

In the acute period pain management relies on intravenous opioids administered as periodic boluses or continuous infusion. Morphine is the most widely used agent, but fentanyl is popular because of its rapid onset, short duration of action, and fewer side effects such as histamine release and peripheral vasodilation. Patient-controlled analgesia (PCA) has been highly effective for older children and adults, because it not only provides better steady- state pain relief but also gives the patient a sense of control.

27. Discuss the management of breakthrough pain and pain related to dressing changes.

It is important to remember that patients have intermittent periods of increased pain known as breakthrough pain. In addition, intense pain may be experienced during dressing changes or therapy. Supplemental pain medication should be given. Unfortunately, any episodes of poorly controlled pain may lead to fear and anxiety before the next procedure. The combination of an anxiolytic agent, such as a benzodiazepine, and an analgesic may better manage the patient's pain experience.

28. How is late pain managed?

In this period, if the gut is working, pain management can be facilitated via oral administration. A preferred long-acting opioid can be given around the clock. A short-acting opioid can be given to accommodate breakthrough pain in addition to the long-acting opioid. Successful management plans have included a cutaneous patch of long-acting opioid applied to healthy nonburned skin. Intravenous opioids are still preferred for any painful procedures such as therapy and dressing changes. Intramuscular analgesia is not recommended because of the unpredictable absorption rates and the need for an additional painful procedure. A good rule of thumb: if the gut works, use it! More interventional modalities may be used if pain control is not sufficient via the oral route.

29. When should rehabilitation begin? What is the role of the trauma nurse?

Rehabilitation should begin on the day of admission. Physical and occupational therapies are of great importance to avoid the formation of contractures. Independently of the patient's general condition, injured upper and lower extremities can be elevated to allow adequate venous drainage and to reduce edema. Passive exercises begin very early after admission, and if the patient is alert and cooperative, he or she is asked to participate in active exercises. Active and passive exercises to maintain range of motion of the joints are continued throughout hospitalization and into the outpatient rehabilitation period.

30. What two important axioms influence rehabilitation?

1. The burn wound will shorten by contraction until it meets an opposing force. Across a flexor surface, the result is a contracture.

2. The position of comfort is the position of contracture. Range-of-motion exercises prevent tendon shortening and restriction of joint motion by burn scar contractures. As patients begin to recover and participate actively in therapy, exercises are designed to increase muscle strength and endurance. A return to activities of daily living frequently takes months of continued rehabilitation.

31. What are the American Burn Association (ABA) recommendations for transferring/transporting patients to a burn center?

1. Partial-thickness burns affecting > 10% TBSA
2. Burns that involve the face, hands, feet, genitalia, perineum, or major joints
3. Third-degree burns in any age group
4. Electrical burns, including lightning
5. Chemical burns
6. Inhalation burns
7. Burn injury in patients with preexisting medical disease that may complicate management, prolong recovery, or affect mortality
8. Any patient with burns and concomitant trauma in which the burn injury poses the greatest risk of morbidity or mortality
9. Burned children in hospitals without qualified personnel or equipment for the care of children
10. Burn injury in patients who require special social, emotional, or long-term rehabilitative intervention

CHEMICAL BURNS

32. What are the common agents that cause chemical burn trauma?

Chemical agents that cause burns are classified by their reactions. In the simplest form, there are four chemical classes: bases, acids, organic compounds, and inorganic agents. However, each of these classes causes tissue damage or burns by more than one chemical reaction.

33. Give common examples of agents in each of these four classes.

CLASS OF AGENT	COMPOUND	COMMON USES
Bases	Alkali: hydroxides, carbonates, caustic sodas of sodium, potassium, ammonium, lithium, barium, and calcium	Oven cleaners, drain cleaners, fertilizers, heavy industrial cleaners, cement or concrete
Acids	Hydrochloric acid (HCL), oxalic acid, sulfuric acid	Bathroom cleaners, acidifiers for swimming pools (HCl), rust removers (oxalic acid); industrial drain cleaners (sulfuric acid)
Organic compounds	Phenols; creosote, petroleum products	Chemical disinfectants (phenols); furniture polishes and gasoline (petroleum)
Inorganic compounds	Sodium, phosphorus, chlorine	Cleaning agents (chlorine)

34. What is the basic pathophysiologic mechanism by which chemical exposure causes burn trauma?

Unlike thermal burns, in which rapid coagulation of proteins results from the hyperthermic activity, chemical burn trauma causes injury by altering tissue proteins, disrupting cellular metabolism, and a wide variety of additional chemical reactions.

35. What factors influence the extent of local and systemic chemical burn injury?

The agent, duration of skin or tissue contact, anatomic location of the burn, and chemical concentration.

36. Which factor can the trauma nurse influence the most and thus reduce the extent of burn trauma?

The duration of the chemical exposure is the easiest factor to manipulate; therefore, it is extremely important that the trauma nurse promptly remove the chemical to prevent further tissue damage. All clothing and jewelry should be removed, and dry chemicals should be brushed off the skin, followed by copious irrigation either in the main treatment area of the emergency department or in a decontamination area.

37. Why is copious irrigation thought to be effective in chemical exposure?

Irrigation is believed to dilute the chemical agent, attenuate the chemical reaction, suppress any elevated tissue metabolism, have an anti-inflammatory action, suppress hygroscopic action, and return tissue pH to normal levels. In addition continued copious irrigation dissipates any heat of dilution that is produced.

38. How do acid burns differ from basic (alkali) burns?

As a general rule alkali burns produce less immediate damage than acids but ultimately cause more tissue destruction by three predominant mechanisms of injury: saponification of fat, extraction of water from cells, and dissolving tissue proteins to form alkaline proteinates, which are involved in further chemical reactions. Neutralizing agents should not be used to treat acid or alkali burns because the heat of the neutralizing may accentuate the severity of injury.

ELECTRICAL BURNS

39. What are the causes of electrical burn trauma?

Causes include lightning strikes, which deliver millions of volts, and electrical current.

40. What are the two types of electrical current?

Direct current (DC): lightning, defibrillators, pacemakers, car battery.

Alternating current (AC): household electrical sources, industrial and high-tension wires.

41. Electrical burns are also defined as low-voltage and high-voltage. What are the major differences?

Low-voltage burns are caused by < 1000 volts, whereas high-voltage injuries are caused by > 1000 volts. Death can occur after exposure to either, but more tissue damage is evident with high-voltage burns.

42. Electrical current travels in the path of least resistance throughout the body. Which body elements have the least resistance and which have the greatest resistance?

Nerves have the least resistance and should be assessed thoroughly in all patients with electrical burn trauma. In particular, the acoustic nerve is often damaged, and hearing should be examined with the initial assessment and throughout the patient's hospitalization. The bones have the greatest resistance to electrical current flow but also generate the most heat and tend to cause necrosis in the deep periosseous tissues.

43. If a patient is exposed to electrical trauma, what are the commonly associated injuries?

Head: blunt trauma, cataracts (immediate or delayed), change or loss of hearing, change in level of consciousness, seizures (immediate or delayed).

Cardiovascular system: asystole, ventricular fibrillation, premature ventricular contractions, atrial fibrillation, S-T and Q-wave abnormalities, bundle-branch blocks, and myocardial infarction. Arterial occlusion due to electrical injury or increased compartmental pressure can develop early or after considerable delay.

Respiratory system: respiratory arrest, aspiration, airway obstruction, pneumothorax, and blunt trauma.

Abdomen and genitourinary system: blunt trauma, renal failure secondary to acute tubular necrosis from large amounts of myoglobin in the urine.

Musculoskeletal and neurologic systems: fractures of long bones and spine, dislocation of joints, blown-off extremities (amputations).

44. Describe the appropriate fluid resuscitation for patients with severe electrical burn trauma.

Fluid resuscitation formulas commonly used for IV fluid resuscitation of patients with thermal burns often underestimate fluid requirements, particularly in patients with deeper, high-voltage electrical burns. Studies have shown that $\geq$ 9 ml/kg/% TBSA of lactated Ringer's solution may be necessary in the first 24 hours to maintain urine output and specific gravity and to reduce myoglobin in the urine. In addition, bicarbonate may be necessary during fluid resuscitation to maintain a urine pH > 7.

BIBLIOGRAPHY

1. Civetta JM, Taylor RW, Kirby RR (eds): Critical Care. Philadelphia, Lippincott-Raven, 1997.
2. Naude GP, Bongard FS, Demetriades D (eds): Trauma Secrets. Philadelphia, Hanley & Belfus, 1999.
3. Oman KS, Koziol-McLain J, Scheetz LJ (eds): Emergency Nursing Secrets. Philadelphia, Hanley & Belfus, 2001.

14. TRAUMA DURING PREGNANCY

Kristopher G. Pidgeon, RN, MSN, CEN, and
Sharon Saunderson Cohen, RN, MSN, CEN, CCRN

1. How common is trauma during pregnancy?

Six to seven percent of all pregnant women experience some sort of trauma, with the greatest frequency in the last trimester. Approximately 0.3–0.4% of pregnant women have traumatic injuries that require hospitalization. Of those injuries, penetrating trauma accounts for as many as 36% of all maternal deaths.

2. What are the morbidity and mortality rates of trauma during pregnancy?

Motor vehicle crashes account for 67% of all major injuries, followed by falls and physical abuse (10–31%). These mechanisms cause placental abruption in as many as 50% of patients with major trauma and as many as 5% of patients with minor trauma. Penetrating wounds injure the fetus in as many as 70% of cases and cause maternal visceral injuries in 19% of cases. Despite the mechanism of injury, the most common cause of fetal death is maternal shock, which is associated with a fetal mortality rate of 80%. Placental abruption is the second most common cause of fetal death, with fetal mortality rates as high as 30–68%. Maternal death results most commonly from brain injury.

3. What is the number-one rule for resuscitation that benefits both mother and fetus?

Resuscitate the mother! Whatever you do for the mother to promote hemodynamic stability also helps the fetus. Survival of the fetus depends on adequate uterine perfusion and delivery of oxygen. The uterine circulation has no autoregulation, which implies that uterine blood flow is related directly to maternal systemic blood pressure, at least until the mother approaches hypovolemic shock. At that point, peripheral vasoconstriction further compromises uterine perfusion. Once obvious shock develops in the mother, the chances of saving the fetus are about 20%.

4. What is the response of the fetus if fetal oxygenation or perfusion is compromised by trauma?

The response of the fetus may include bradycardia or tachycardia, a decrease in the baseline variability of the heart rate, absence of normal accelerations in the heart rate, or recurrent decelerations. An abnormal fetal heart rate may be the first indication of an important disruption in fetal homeostasis.

5. During trauma resuscitation, fetal evaluation should begin with what?

Fetal evaluation should begin with auscultation of fetal heart tones and continuous recording of the fetal heart rate.

6. What is the normal range for fetal heart tones (FHTs)?

FHTs may be heard with a fetoscope at approximately 20 weeks' gestation and by an ultrasound device at 10–14 weeks' gestation. Auscultate for 2 minutes. The fetal heart rate is normally 120–160 beats per minute (bpm). A sustained fetal heart rate < 110 bpm is considered bradycardic. A sustained fetal heart rate > 160 bpm is considered tachycardic.

7. Uterine contractions are common after major or minor trauma. Explain their cause and significance.

Trauma to the uterus (direct or indirect) can also injure the myometrium and destabilize decidual lysosomes, releasing arachidonic acid that can cause uterine contractions and perhaps induce premature labor. Because of the higher risk for premature labor, most pregnant trauma patients are admitted for treatment of injuries and fetal monitoring.

8. What signs and symptoms during assessment of pregnant trauma patients may indicate premature labor?

In conscious patients, premature labor may be noted by uterine contractions > 6/hour; back pain; and clear or bloody vaginal drainage. In unconscious patients, fetal monitoring is needed to monitor contractions.

9. Many maternal physiologic changes during pregnancy may directly affect the assessment and treatment plan. What are some of these physiologic changes?

SYSTEM	MATERNAL PHYSIOLOGIC CHANGE	NURSING CONSIDERATIONS	COMMENTS
Cardiac	↑ CO and blood volume	Hypervolemic and hemo-diluted state may be protective of mother during hemorrhage	40% of maternal blood volume may be lost before signs/symptoms of maternal shock appear
Thoracic	As uterus enlarges, diaphragm rises about 4 cm and diameter of chest increases by 2 cm; substantial angle increases by 50%	Care needed in doing thoracic procedures such as thoracostomies	
Pulmonary	↑ TV and FRC, ↑ oxygen consumption by 20% Hyperventilation as much as 50% at term	Supplemental oxygen is always indicated pCO_2 falls to 30–32 mmHg with a slight ↓ in plasma bicarbonate	Supply of oxygen must meet demands
Renal	↑ GFR, ↓ BUN and creatinine	Kidneys enlarge as early as 10th week	May be more prone to injury
Neurologic	↓ Anesthetic requirements by 25–40%	Loss of consciousness can occur at "sedative" doses	Decreased level of consciousness may be first sign of maternal shock
Gastrointestinal	Decrease in gastric motility Decrease in competency of gastroesophageal sphincter Increase in uterine size displaces intestines upward	Increased risk of aspiration Decreased reliability of abdominal examination	

CO = cardiac output, TV = tidal volume, FRC = forced residual capacity, pCO_2 = partial pressure of carbon dioxide, GFR = glomerular filtration rate, BUN = blood urea nitrogen.

10. How do the priorities for treatment of traumatic injuries differ in pregnant and nonpregnant patients?

The priorities are the same. As with any patient, pregnant or not, the initial assessment addresses the ACBCDs: airway, cervical spine, breathing, circulation, and disability (neurologic status).

11. Which position is best for pregnant trauma patients?

Pregnant patients beyond 20 weeks' gestation should not be kept in the supine position. Uterine displacement should be to the left. This displacement can be attained by tilting the backboard and supporting it with a towel roll or two to the left or by manual displacement. Such a position prevents aortocaval compression and the subsequent drop in maternal cardiac output.

12. Is there a role for pneumatic antishock garments (PASG) or military antishock trousers (MAST) in pregnant trauma patients?

Yes. PASG or MAST may be used to stabilize lower extremity fractures and possibly control hemorrhage in these areas. Inflation of the abdominal compartment of the PASG/MAST should be avoided because it compromises uteroplacental blood flow.

13. What lab studies should be considered for pregnant trauma patients? Why?

Complete blood count (CBC). Pregnancy-induced leukocytosis peaks to levels of 12,000–18,000/mm^3 during the third trimester. CBC also provide the baseline hemoglobin and hematocrit levels of the mother.

Rhesus (Rh) blood group assesses the need to administer RhoGAM if the mother is Rh-negative. If both father and mother are negative, RhoGAM does not need to be given.

Quantitative beta human chorionic gonadotropin (β-hCG) allows an additional determination of gestational age (along with the maternal history and ultrasound). It also determines whether the patient is actually pregnant!

The **Kleihauer-Betke test** is used to detect fetal-to-maternal hemorrhage, which may occur in as many as 30% of all major traumas.

Coagulation panel and D-dimer assay assess for coagulopathies. The placenta releases thromboplastin when it is injured. When thromboplastin gets into the maternal circulation, disseminated intravascular coagulation (DIC) can develop rapidly.

14. Is it safe to perform diagnostic peritoneal lavage (DPL) in pregnant trauma patients?

Yes. DPL should be done above the umbilicus with an open technique.

15. Which noninvasive diagnostic test is used to evaluate the abdomen of pregnant trauma patients?

Ultrasonography is used to assess the abdomen for free fluid or free air as well as to evaluate the fetus. In addition, it is safe for the fetus and in most institutions does not require the mother to be moved out of the area where resuscitation is performed.

16. What injuries can occur specifically during pregnancy after a traumatic event? What signs and symptoms may raise suspicion of the diagnosis?

DIAGNOSIS	ASSESSMENT FINDINGS	COMMENTS
Abruptio placentae	Fetal distress on monitoring; tense abdomen with uterine hypotonia, maternal hypertension or hypotension, ultrasonographic evidence of abruption	May be delayed for as long as 24–48 hours
Uterine rupture	Two abdominal masses: one is the uterus and one the fetus	Fetal death is common. Control of hemorrhage is imperative for maternal survival.
Amniotic fluid embolus	Sudden onset of dyspnea, hypoxemia, and tachypnea; can be followed by ARDS and DIC	Treatment, given in ICU, includes ventilator and supportive care

Table continued on following page

DIAGNOSIS	ASSESSMENT FINDINGS	COMMENTS
Premature labor	Tense abdomen, contractions noted on fetal monitoring	Because abruptio placentae is also associated with contractions, assume that it is present.
Premature rupture of membranes (PROM)	Clear to bloody fluid present on pelvic examination; check fluid pH with nitrazine paper	Vaginal excretions have pH of 5–6, whereas pH of amniotic fluid is > 7. Less accurate pH with nitrazine in presence of blood

ARDS = acute respiratory distress syndrome, DIC = disseminated intravascular coagulation.

17. What is a simple method to assess the pregnant trauma patient for contractions?

The quickest and easiest way is to place your hand on the patient's pregnant belly and feel for constant or intermittent rigidity. This technique also allows the trauma nurse to displace the abdomen to the left if it has not already been done.

18. Why is it important to assess and document the fundal height early in the evaluation of a pregnant trauma patient?

Initial and ongoing fundal height assessment is imperative to assess any increase in fundal height. Because of the potential for loss of up to 40% of maternal blood volume before signs and symptoms of shock are noted, ongoing abdominal hemorrhage can be detected at an earlier point by increases in fundal height.

19. Can a pregnant trauma patient receive tetanus prophylaxis?

Yes. Like all treatment options, contraindications need to be assessed (e.g., allergies), but pregnancy is not considered a contraindication. Most often the benefit of vaccination outweighs any risks.

20. What pain medications are safe to administer in pregnancy?

Category A or B analgesics (e.g., acetaminophen, meperidine, morphine, fentanyl, hydrocodone) are first choices. Other options may include category C drugs (e.g., codeine, ibuprofen, salicylates, indomethacin), which should be used with caution in pregnancy. A bit of caution should be noted when salicylate-containing analgesics are used in trauma patients, who may be at greater risk for bleeding.

21. Is it acceptable to perform a postmortem cesarean section?

Yes. Postmortem cesarean sections have a 15% success rate. The most important factors are probably fetus-related. If the fetus is older than 29 weeks and weighs more than 1000 gm, survival is obviously improved, especially if maternal oxygenation and perfusion are adequate.

BIBLIOGRAPHY

1. Cardona VD: The pregnant trauma patient. In Trauma Nursing: From Resuscitation Through Rehabilitation, 2nd ed. Philadelphia, W.B. Saunders, 1994.
2. Chang AK: Pregnancy, trauma. E-Med J 2(8), 2001.
3. Pearlman MD, et al: Blunt trauma during pregnancy. N Engl J Med 323:1609–1613, 1990.

15. PEDIATRIC TRAUMA

Cindy A. Garlesky, MSN, ARNP, CEN

1. What anatomic and physiologic features affect a child's response to trauma?

ANATOMIC/PHYSIOLOGIC FEATURES	CLINICAL IMPLICATIONS
Large tongue	Easily obstructs airway
High metabolic rate influences oxygen and glucose consumption	Administer high-flow supplemental oxygen; monitor glucose levels
Large body surface area and less mature thermoregulatory mechanism increases risk for hypothermia	Monitor body temperature and keep child warm
Relatively unprotected abdominal organs	Abdominal organs easily injured in blunt trauma without visible signs of injury
Diaphragm excursion impaired by pressure from distended stomach	Insert nasogastric/orogastric tube to reduce distention
Increased heart rate can reflect altered cardiac output as well as fear, fever, and pain	Assess circulation and monitor capillary refill, central vs. peripheral pulses, color, skin temperature, and level of consciousness
Circulating volume = 80 ml/kg	Small blood or fluid losses can compromise circulation

2. What interventions can reduce the risk of hypothermia in the pediatric trauma patient?
- Increase the ambient temperature of the trauma room.
- Remove all wet clothing or wet items.
- Keep the child covered with a warm blanket or warming device.
- Use overhead warming lights.
- Administer warm intravenous fluids.
- Monitor body temperature on arrival and routinely thereafter.

3. What is the most common type of traumatic injury in children?
Approximately 80–90% of all pediatric injuries result from blunt trauma. Common mechanisms of injury include motor vehicle crashes (child as passenger), vehicle vs. pedestrian collisions, falls from heights, and bicycle crashes.

4. Describe Waddell's triad.
Waddell's triad is a common pattern of blunt injury in children who are struck by motor vehicles. It results in multisystem injuries. The constellation of injuries depends on the physical size of the child and the vehicle involved. Most commonly, the triad includes chest or abdominal injuries, head injuries, and lower extremity fractures.

5. What are the three most common causes of death in pediatric trauma patients?
- Head injury
- Blood loss
- Multisystem organ failure

Apply the following scenario to questions 6–13: A 3-year-old boy is found on the ground after falling from a third-story window. His color is pale; he has no abnormal airway sounds or increased work of breathing. He does not respond to verbal stimuli but makes grunting sounds, opens his eyes, and flexes his extremities when the intravenous line is started. Vital signs include spontaneous respiration of 24 breaths/minute, heart rate of 160 beats/minute, and capillary refill of 3 seconds.

6. What are the priorities in terms of assessment and intervention?
Interventions should follow the primary survey assessment of A, B, C, and D:

1. The first priority is to assess for (A) airway patency while maintaining cervical spine stabilization and to initiate interventions to maintain airway patency.

2. Once a patent airway has been established and the cervical spine is stabilized, the second step is to assess adequacy and effectiveness of (B) breathing and intervene as indicated.

3. Once adequate breathing is established, the third step is to assess adequacy and effectiveness of (C) circulation and intervene as indicated.

4. The final step in the primary survey includes a brief neurologic assessment to determine the degree of (D) disability.

7. List the possible interventions to maintain a patent airway.
• Jaw thrust
• Suction
• Oral or nasopharyngeal airway
• Laryngeal mask airway (LMA)
• Endotracheal intubation
• Cricothyrotomy (rarely indicated in children younger than 8 years of age)

8. Describe the clinical presentation of a child with tension pneumothorax.
• Sudden decompensation in clinical status.
• Severe respiratory distress with dyspnea.
• Shift of the point of maximal impulse (PMI). A shift to the left of the nipple line indicates right-sided tension; a shift to the right of the nipple line indicates left-sided tension.
• Circulatory compromise as the heart and great vessels are pushed over.
• Decreased or absent chest expansion.
• Diminished or absent breath sounds.
• Distended neck veins and tracheal shifts are rarely seen in children because of their short neck.

9. Describe your plan for assessment and treatment of circulatory status.
The increased heart rate, pale skin color, delayed capillary refill, and altered level of consciousness reflect circulatory compromise due to blood loss. Assess for any obvious signs of bleeding, and apply pressure as needed. Obtain two large-bore vascular access devices, and prepare to administer a 20-ml/kg bolus of warmed crystalloid. Reassess after bolus is administered. Consider the mechanism of injury and the areas of the body that may be bleeding. Possibilities include pulmonary, cardiac, and/or abdominal injuries as well as pelvic or femoral fractures.

10. How should you obtain the boy's weight to calculate the fluid bolus?
A length-based resuscitation tape (also known as a pediatric resuscitation tape) is a simple tool to measure the length of the child (from the top of the head to the heel) and approximate his kilogram weight. These tapes provide drug doses, amounts of fluid boluses, and equipment sizes for children weighing between 3 and 34 kg.

11. What is the boy's score on the Glasgow Coma Scale (GCS)?

The boy's score is 8, as calculated from the GCS:

EYE OPENING		VERBAL RESPONSE		BEST MOTOR RESPONSE	
				6*	Obeys verbal commands
		5	Oriented, appropriate sounds	5	Localizes pain, purposeful
4	Spontaneous	4	Disoriented	4	Withdraws (from pain)
3	To command	3	Inappropriate sounds	3	Flexion
2	To pain	2	Incomprehensible sounds	2	Extension
1	No response	1	No response	1	No response

* Not applicable in children younger than 1 year of age.

12. What does a GCS ≤ 8 indicate?

A GCS ≤ 8 is one criterion for intubation. It indicates severe neurologic injury and increases the risks for loss of an adequate airway and development of increased intracranial pressure and cerebral edema.

13. Describe an intervention to facilitate atraumatic intubation.

Rapid-sequence induction intubation (RSI) involves the use of combinations of medications, including sedative-hyponotics, analgesics, and neuromuscular blocking agents, to sedate and anesthetize a responsive or unresponsive child before intubation. It reduces the physiologic response to intubation and the risk of causing trauma during the procedure. In pediatric patients, lidocaine and atropine are commonly added as presedation medications to reduce stimulation of the gag reflex and the associated bradycardia. The hemodynamic status is a major factor in determining the medication combination used for RSI.

14. Describe blunt abdominal injuries in children.

Common mechanisms of abdominal injury in children include seat belts, handlebars, and direct blows. The most prevalent abdominal injuries in children include perforation of the bowel, liver, and spleen. Diagnosis of these injuries is often delayed, especially in children less than five years of age where the initial abdominal examination is often difficult and may be unreliable.

15. How are abdominal injuries treated?

Compared with adults, very few children require immediate laparotomy. Conservative (nonoperative) management of abdominal injuries is the treatment of choice in pediatric trauma patients unless the child has continued unstable vitals signs, falling hemoglobin and hematocrit despite treatment, pneumoperitoneum, peritonitis on exam, bladder rupture, rectal laceration, or penetrating injuries.

16. What is the appropriate pain assessment tool for a preschool child?

The Faces Tool is recommended for children between the ages of 3 and 12 years. It consists of 6 cartoon faces ranging from a smiling face for "no pain" to a fearful face for "worst pain." In addition, the Face, Legs, Activity, Cry, and Consolability (FLACC) scale can be used for children between the ages of 2 months and 7 years. This scale involves assessment of the five FLACC parameters, using a scale to rate the pain between 0 and 2 for each parameter. The Numeric Scale for pain assessment is preferred to determine pain level in adolescents. One end of the line is 0 for "no pain," and the other end is 5 for "worst pain." All children can be assessed for pain using behavioral cues and physiologic signs. Behavioral cues of pain may include crying, grimacing, decreased activity, altered sleep pattern, and diaphoresis. Physiologic signs of pain include increased heart rate, increased blood pressure, increased respiratory rate, and increased body temperature. Pain assessment is the "fifth vital sign" and is an essential component of assessment for all children.

17. How does a child's cognitive development affect reaction to and perception of pain?

Infants may have a memory of painful events but respond primarily to parental displays of anxiety. Toddlers are more egocentric and may react to the loss of control or autonomy if they are restrained or unable to move; this reaction may be compounded by stranger anxiety if parents are not present. Preschoolers often react to pain as a punishment to something they did and intensely fear bodily injury, especially if blood is visible to them. School-aged children often react to pain out of fear of body mutilation and loss of control; however, they are beginning to understand the relationship of cause and effect. The invincible adolescent may not display pain behaviors because of fear of embarrassment and loss of control.

18. Describe methods for acute pain management in pediatric trauma patients.

The management of acute pain in children includes both nonpharmacologic and pharmacologic interventions. Nonpharmacologic interventions may include distraction (e.g., music, videos, toys, breathing techniques, imagery); touch and tactile stimulation (e.g., massage, application of cold and warmth, physical therapy); immobilization, splinting, and elevation; and alternative therapies such as acupuncture. Pharmacologic interventions include nonopioid medications (e.g., acetaminophen, salicylates, nonsteroidal anti-inflammatory drugs), opioids (e.g., morphine, meperidine), inhaled agents (e.g., nitrous oxide), local anesthetics and blocks, and adjunctive agents (e.g., sedatives, anxiolytics). Pain management of pediatric trauma patients most commonly includes combinations of nonpharmacologic and pharmacologic interventions that minimize the child's experience of pain, facilitate accurate assessment, and promote the healing process.

19. When should a pediatric trauma patient be immobilized on a backboard?

Spinal immobilization should be initiated on arrival and maintained until the cervical spine is cleared in any child who sustains a mechanism of injury suspicious for spinal injury, who is unconscious, who has a major head injury, or who is developmentally unreliable.

20. Describe the procedure for spinal immobilization in pediatric trauma patients.

- Assess peripheral circulation and motor and sensory (CMS) status.
- Manually stabilize the cervical spine until the child is completely secured to the rigid surface.
- Initiate cervical immobilization with a collar, towel rolls, or head blocks.
- Log roll the child onto a rigid surface while maintaining cervical stabilization. Consider use of a shoulder roll for children less than 8 years of age because of the large occiput.
- Secure the child's body onto the rigid surface, taping or strapping over the bony prominences. Avoid constriction across the chest wall and abdomen.
- Secure the head. Tape or strap across the forehead only. Avoid taping to the lower jaw. If using tape, place the tape directly on the skin surface.
- Assess CMS.

21. Describe considerations for facilitating family presence during pediatric trauma resuscitation.

Facilitating family presence during invasive procedures and resuscitation has gained recognition in recent years. Many studies promote the acceptance of this practice. The family is the main source of support and comfort for a child. Considerations for involving the family should include the following:

1. Provide the family with the opportunity to be present in the treatment or resuscitation area.

2. Appoint one staff member to remain with the family.

3. Prepare the family for what they will hear, see, and smell.
4. Allow parents to see and touch their child.
5. Reassess the family frequently.

22. How are submersion injuries defined in children?

Submersion injuries in children include both drowning and near-drowning events. The term *drowning* refers to death by asphyxiation after submersion in water or other liquids. The term *near-drowning* refers to submersion injuries in which the victim survives for at least the first 24 hours after the event.

23. What body systems are most affected by submersion injuries?

Although submersion injuries involve both pulmonary and neurologic complications, generally the anoxic insult to the brain is primarily responsible for the major hemodynamic changes. The severity of the neurologic complications may be related to a number of factors, including the duration of the submersion, the temperature of the immersion liquid, and the time elapsed before effective cardiopulmonary resuscitation was provided. The severity of the effects on the pulmonary system depends on whether the event is defined as a wet or dry drowning. **Wet drowning** occurs as the child attempts to breathe underwater and the pulmonary system is flooded with aspirated liquid. Wet drowning results in pulmonary hypertension and surfactant wash-out, which progresses to the development of atelectasis, acute respiratory distress syndrome, and pulmonary edema. This process has been termed *secondary drowning*. **Dry drowning** occurs when the child suffers laryngospasm and aspirates very little of the submersion liquid.

24. List the potential complications of pediatric trauma.

- Hypovolemic shock
- Increased intracranial pressure (ICP)
- Septic shock
- Meningitis
- Neurogenic shock
- Compartment syndrome
- Tension pneumothorax
- Skin breakdown
- Hemothorax
- Peritonitis
- Acute respiratory distress syndrome (ARDS)
- Syndrome of inappropriate antidiuretic hormone (SIADH)
- Pneumonia
- Diabetes insipidus
- Pulmonary emboli
- Disseminated intravascular coagulation (DIC)
- Atelectasis
- Gastrointestinal bleed

25. What controversies are involved in the management of pediatric submersion victims?

Management of submersion victims focuses on two phases of care:

Phase one is the stabilization time, which includes well-established practices such as initial assessment and management of the ABCDs, assessment of cervical spine, metabolic support for nutrition and seizure control, ongoing neurologic exams, pulmonary management, and management of ICP.

Phase two revolves around ongoing maintenance of the child and prevention of secondary complications. The major controversies in care exist in this phase of management and involve the use of barbiturate coma, hypothermia, or steroids.

26. Discuss the role of rehabilitation for head-injured children.

Rehabilitation for head-injured children focuses on dealing with motor, neurologic, and psychological impairments after injury. The goals are to return the child to his or her maximal potential and to improve the child's readjustment at home and school. The recovery period for motor and sensory injuries is reported to vary from 9 months to 1 year. However, the neurologic, psychological, behavioral, and emotional deficits of the head injury may extend beyond several years.

27. What are the differences between enteral and parenteral feeding in pediatric trauma patients?

ENTERAL FEEDING	TOTAL PARENTERAL FEEDING
More physiologically normal	Insertion site is common infection source
Helps to normalize gastric pH	Tolerated by children who do not tolerate enteral feeds
Causes fewer electrolyte imbalances	Higher risk for electrolyte imbalance and fluid shifts
Aids in prevention of stress ulcer	Risk of pneumothorax during insertion
Greater risk of aspiration	May alter liver function tests (LFTs)
Diarrhea may result	Glucose intolerance may result

28. What is the prognosis for children suffering cardiopulmonary arrest after sustaining blunt trauma?

The prognosis for children in cardiopulmonary arrest or children with systolic blood pressures < 50 mmHg is poor. In the few children who survive (< 1%), functional outcome is dismal.

29. What are the main types of child maltreatment?
- Neglect
- Physical abuse
- Emotional abuse
- Sexual abuse

30. What information helps to screen all children for suspected maltreatment?
- The history does not match the injury.
- The history does not match the developmental abilities of the child.
- The child has suspicious markings or injuries.
- There is an inconsistent or vague account of the event.
- There is an unreasonable delay in seeking medical attention.

31. Which states have laws that mandate reporting of child maltreatment?

All 50 states have passed laws to protect children by requiring mandatory reporting of suspected or known child abuse and neglect.

BIBLIOGRAPHY

1. American Academy of Pediatrics: Pediatric Education for Prehospital Providers. Boston, Jones & Bartlett, 2000.
2. Beyda DH: Childhood submersion injuries. J Emerg Nurs 24(2):140–144, 1998.
3. Canty T Sr, Canty T Jr, Brown C: Injuries of the gastrointestinal tract from blunt trauma in children. J Trauma 46:234–230, 1999.
4. Eckle N, MacLean SL: Assessment of family-centered care policies and practices for pediatric patients in nine U.S. emergency departments. J Emerg Nurs 27:238–245, 2001.

5. Emergency Nurses Association: Emergency Nursing Pediatric Course: Provider Manual. Park Ridge, IL; Emergency Nurses Association, 1998.
6. Franck LS, Greenberg CS, Stevens B: Pain assessment in infants and children. Pediatr Clin North Am 47:487–512, 2000.
7. Golianu B, Krane EJ, Galloway KS, Yaster M: Pediatric acute pain management. Pediatr Clin North Am 47:559–587, 2000.
8. Li G, Tang N, Scala C, et al: Cardiopulmonary resuscitation in pediatric trauma patients: Survival and functional outcome. J Trauma 47:1–7, 1999.
9. McQuillan KA, et al (eds): Trauma Nursing: From Resuscitation through Rehabilitation, 3rd ed. Philadelphia, W.B. Saunders, 2002.
10. Mikhail J (ed): Advanced Practice in Acute and Critical Care. AACN Clin Issues 10(1):10–21, 1999.
11. Meyer M, Burd RS: The trauma top ten: The top 10 things to evaluate in children with suspected blunt abdominal injuries. J Trauma Nurs 7(4):98–102, 2000.
12. Reece RM, Ludwig S (eds): Child Abuse: Medical Diagnosis and Management. Philadelphia, Lippincott Williams & Wilkins, 2001.
13. Youngblut JS, Singer LT, Poyer C, et al: Effects of pediatric head trauma for children, parents and families. Crit Care Nurs Clin North Am 12:227–235, 2000.

16. GERIATRIC TRAUMA

Patricia A. Manion, RN, MS, CCRN

1. What is the most common cause of death due to trauma in the geriatric population?
The most common cause of death from trauma is motor vehicle crashes (MVCs) in the 65- to 74-year-old population; falls are the most common cause of death from trauma in the 75 and older age group.

2. What common patterns are seen in MVCs among the elderly?
MVCs among the elderly tend to occur during the day, in good weather, close to home, and at intersections. In 80% of MVCs, the elderly driver is considered "at fault."

3. Is alcohol abuse a common problem among the elderly?
About 3 million of the 10 million alcoholics in the United States are over the age of 60. In 1999, 9% of all drivers aged 55–69 years who were involved in fatal crashes were intoxicated (blood alcohol concentrations $\geq$ 0.10 gm/dl). In the 70+ age group, 4% were intoxicated.

4. Do geriatric patients have the expected tachycardic response to hypovolemia?
In general, yes. However, a number of factors can prevent the expected tachycardia in the geriatric trauma patients with hypovolemia. The patient may be taking beta blockers, which prevent the increase in heart rate associated with sympathetic nervous system response to hypovolemia. The patient may have preexisting disease of the sinus node that prevents an increase in the sinus rate or disease of the atrioventricular node that prevents impulses from reaching the ventricles. Geriatric patients also may have an acute process, such as acute myocardial ischemia or infarction, that affects the sinus node or conduction system.

5. Is aggressive fluid resuscitation a safe intervention in geriatric trauma patients?
Yes, with precautions. The cardiovascular changes that occur with aging include increasing ventricular wall thickness, decreasing compliance, loss of vascular elasticity, increased vascular resistance, and decreased sensitivity of the baroreceptors. The older patient may have preexisting comorbidities such as diabetes mellitus, hypertension, myocardial infarction, or heart failure. Resuscitation of the elderly patient should be guided by early placement of intravenous lines for hemodynamic monitoring.

6. Why are rib fractures more dangerous in geriatric patients?
Elderly patients in MVCs are at increased risk of sustaining rib fractures, and these injuries are highly associated with fatality. The effects of aging on the respiratory system include a decrease in the number of functioning alveoli, loss of elasticity of the alveoli and chest wall, decreased vital capacity, and decreased cough effectiveness. Elderly patients may have preexisting chronic obstructive pulmonary disease and often have chronic colonization of the upper airways with enteric bacteria, which can predispose to pneumonia.

7. What are two important questions to ask after an elderly patient sustains a fall?
1. What caused the fall?
2. What are the injuries?

8. List the common pathophysiologic reasons for falls in the elderly.
• Syncopal events due to bradydysrhythmias or tachydysrhythmias
• Anemia related to gastrointestinal bleeds

- Transient ischemic attacks (TIAs) or strokes
- Postural hypotension related to certain medications or physiologic effects of aging
- Effects of alcohol
- Hypoglycemia or hyperglycemia
- Chronic subdural hematoma
- Pathologic hip fractures
- Peripheral neuropathies related to diabetes or renal failure
- Acute myocardial infarction

9. What prior therapies should be continued in admitted trauma patients?

PRIOR THERAPIES	EXAMPLES
Pharmacologic agents	Cardiovascular: antiarrhythmics, angiotensin-converting enzyme (ACE) inhibitors, digoxin, nitrates, diuretics
	Hormone replacement therapy: estrogen, thyroid, insulin
	Glaucoma medications
	Asthma medications and inhaler
	Antiseizure medications
Electrical therapies	Pacemakers
	Transcutaneous electrical nerve stimulation (TENS) units
	Implanted cardioverter defibrillator devices
	Hearing aids
	Continuous positive airway pressure (CPAP) and biphasic positive airway pressure (BiPAP)
Assistive devices	Walkers
	Canes
	Prostheses
Medical interventions	Dialysis
	Home oxygen therapy
	Intermittent inotropic therapy for heart failure

10. What are the most common infections in geriatric patients after traumatic injury?
Pneumonia and line sepsis.

11. Why are geriatric patients with orthopedic injuries at increased risk for poor wound healing and infections?
The risk of complications is increased because of preexisting vascular insufficiency, diabetes, immunocompromise, osteopenia, and poor nutrition.

12. List special considerations in the treatment of pain in elderly trauma patients.
1. Elderly people are more sensitive to the therapeutic and toxic effects of analgesics.

2. The use of nonsteroidal anti-inflammatory medications is more likely to cause peptic ulcer disease and gastrointestinal bleeding.

3. The decrease in lean body mass, increase in proportion of body fat, and decrease in water affects the distribution of drugs. Morphine, which is water-soluble, has a lower volume of distribution, a more rapid onset of action and an increased peak concentration in the elderly. These high peak concentrations may increase toxicity. Therefore, dosing should begin at 50–75% of recommended dose and titrated on the basis of patient response. Fentanyl is fat-soluble and, therefore, may be distributed more widely, have a delayed onset of action, and accumulate with repeated dosing.

4. Because of decreased muscle mass and possible decreased perfusion, intramuscular dosing is to be avoided.

5. Age- and disease-related changes in the liver and kidneys may increase the risk for accumulation and toxicity of drugs with a long half-life. Opioid analgesics with short half-lives, such as morphine, hydromorphone, and oxycodone, are often better choices in the elderly.

6. Meperidine should be avoided in the elderly because it produces a toxic metabolite, normeperidine, which has a long half-life and can lead to central nervous system disturbances ranging from dysphoria to seizures.

7. The elderly are at increased risk for the constipation that often results from opioid use because of concomitant decrease in gastric and bowel motility.

13. Is it important to differentiate between dementia and delirium in elderly trauma patients? What is the difference?

It is very important to differentiate between dementia and delirium. **Dementia** is an impairment of memory accompanied by changes in personality, abstract thinking, or other higher cortical functions. Dementia is a chronic condition with gradual onset. Causes of dementia include decreased perfusion to the brain (stroke, atherosclerosis), Alzheimer's disease, old head injury, chronic alcoholism, or nutritional deficits. **Delirium** is an abrupt change in the level of consciousness and is a medical emergency. Delirium may result from acute head injury, sepsis, adverse drug reactions, and hypoxemia.

14. Which common laboratory values are "normally abnormal" in geriatric patients?

Common Changes in Laboratory Values in Geriatric Patients

INCREASED	UNCHANGED	DECREASED
Blood urea nitrogen	Sedimentation rate	Albumin
Glucose	Hemoglobin	Calcium
Fibrinogen	Prothrombin time, partial thromboplastin time	Creatinine clearance
Alkaline phosphatase	Electrolytes	Phosphorus
Uric acid	Aspartate aminotransferase	
	Creatinine	
	White blood cell count	

15. Do geriatric patients have a higher mortality rate after major trauma?

Yes. The case fatality rate for hospitalized older trauma patients is between 15% and 30% compared with 4–8% for younger patients.

16. List three requirements for admission of a geriatric patient to acute inpatient rehabilitation.

1. Ability to complete 3 hours of therapy per day.
2. Ability to participate in the therapy (i.e., cooperate and follow directions).
3. Potential for independent or semi-independent living on discharge.

BIBLIOGRAPHY

1. Emergency Nurses Association: Trauma Nursing Core Course, 5th ed. Des Plaines, IL, Emergency Nurses Association, 2000.
2. Frankenfield MS, et al: Age-related differences in the metabolic response to injury. J Trauma 48:49–57, 2000.
3. Higgins JP, Wright SW, Wrenn KD: Alcohol, the elderly, and motor vehicle crashes. Am J Emerg Med 14:265–267, 1996.
4. Hudak CM, Gallo BM, Morton PG: Critical Care Nursing, 7th ed. Philadelphia, Lippincott, 1998.
5. Koval KJ: Treatment of Fractures in the Elderly. 21st Annual Trauma Seminar, Orthopaedic Course Reports. Available at www.Medscape.com.

6. Lakhani N: Alcohol use among community-dwelling elderly people: A review of the literature. J Adv Nurs 25:1227–1232, 1997.
7. McGwin G, et al: Long-term survival in the elderly after trauma. J Trauma 49:470–476, 2000.
8. National Highway Safety and Transportation Authority: Traffic Safety Facts 1999: Older Population. Available at www.nhsta.gov.
9. Pasero CL: How aging affects pain management. Am J Nurs 98:12, 1998.
10. Springhouse Corporation: Handbook or Geriatric Drug Therapy. Springhouse, PA, Springhouse Corporation, 2000.
11. Wang SC: An aging population: Fragile, handle with care. Available at www-nrd.nhsta.dot.gov.

17. DOMESTIC VIOLENCE AND ABUSE

Stephen M. Cohen, MS, PA-C, EdD (c)

1. Define domestic violence.

State laws define domestic violence. Clinicians must read and understand the state application of domestic violence law to be effective in practice.

In general, domestic violence can be defined as actual or threatened emotional, physical, psychological, financial, or sexual abuse of a person by a spouse, former spouse, partner, former partner, adult relative, or parent of a minor child. Abuse may include threats, harm, injury, harassment, control, terrorism, or damage to living beings or property. The clinician also should consider domestic violence as including violence toward the elderly and children. In the case of the elderly and children, we add the category of neglect as a type of violence.

2. What are the basic facts about domestic violence?
- Battering is a pattern, a reign of force and terror.
- Only the perpetrator has the ability to stop the violence.
- It may take up to 7 incidents before a victim leaves a violent living arrangement.
- Approximately 2000 women a year (in the United States) die before they leave.
- Drinking and drug use do not cause domestic violence.
- Batterers should never be given custody or unsupervised visitation of children. A connection between missing and battered children and domestic violence–related divorce is possible.
- Batterers have excellent impulse control. They beat only their partner.

3. How common is domestic violence?

Battering is extremely common. Estimates have shown that as many as 1 in 3 emergency room patients are victims of domestic violence. Nearly one-half of all child abuse victims can relate a story of parental domestic violence also. One in 5 women presenting with a sexually transmitted disease may be victims of domestic violence.

4. What is the role of trauma, emergency, and critical care nurses in domestic violence forensics?

The nurse's role is not only to provide physical and emotional care to patients but also to help preserve the chain of evidence collection (chain of custody). Nursing personnel are also in an excellent position to collaborate with physicians, physician assistants, social services, law enforcement, and courts to help develop guidelines for forensic evidence collection and documentation. All nurses exposed to outpatient care should become familiar with the concepts and skills of evidence collection and photographic and written documentation.

5. Discuss the connection between pregnancy and domestic violence.

Partner violence is positively related to pregnancy; 17% of pregnant women are battered. Family stress and multiple, closely spaced pregnancies are possible correlates of domestic violence during pregnancy. A woman is more likely to be a victim when pregnant than when not pregnant. Pregnant women are at risk for intentional trauma and pose unique challenges for care. Injury caused by domestic violence is associated with the greatest risk of obstetric complications. Twenty-five to 45% of battered women have been battered in pregnancy, increasing the incidence of miscarriage, preterm labor, and low birth weight.

6. Is there any connection between substance abuse in women and domestic violence?

Yes. Women who are substance users are more likely to be victims of domestic violence than nonsubstance users.

7. What is the connection between child abuse and domestic violence?

It is estimated that more than 50% of the victims of domestic violence were also victims of abuse as a child. In addition, it appears that if domestic spousal abuse occurs in the home, children in the home are more likely to be abused.

8. How does clinical forensics apply to domestic violence?

Clinical forensics is the specialized application of scientific and clinical medical knowledge to legal and criminal matters such as domestic violence. Many domestic violence police investigation units use clinical forensic information and personnel for investigation and victim support.

9. Can domestic violence present as trauma?

Yes. Many so-called accidents, such as falls, are the result of domestic violence. Patients presenting with trauma unrelated to motor vehicle crashes, especially assault-related trauma, should prompt inquiry about the possibility of injury by a known partner. Many injuries sustained in a single-vehicle crash, either as driver or passenger, are also caused by domestic violence. It is appropriate to ask all trauma patients about the possibility of causation by another person.

10. Can domestic violence present as something other than trauma?

Yes. It is not uncommon to ascertain in shelters and counseling that the initial presentation to a medical clinic or emergency department was for a problem other than trauma. Among the most commonly reported problems are headache, pelvic pain, abdominal pain, dizziness, sexually transmitted disease, joint pain, acute intoxication or drug overdose, and gastrointestinal illness. Victims of domestic violence have more lifetime, non–trauma-related surgery than nonvictims. Battering accounts for 25% of female suicide attempts. Forty percent of battered women are raped by their partners. Domestic violence is also a frequent precipitant of psychiatric emergencies.

11. Why is domestic violence an important issue in community health?

Important community problems can be directly linked to domestic violence. Eighty percent of runaways are from abusive homes. Juvenile delinquents are four times more likely to come from abusive homes. Sixty-three percent of all boys aged 11–20 years who are arrested for homicide killed their mothers' assaulters. In 50% of cases, both child abuse and domestic violence are present in the same home. Children from these homes are 1000 times more likely to abuse as adults.

12. What does the Joint Commission for Accreditation of Healthcare Organizations (JCAHO) say about institution policy and procedure regarding domestic violence?

1. Hospitals must have policies for the identification, evaluation, management, and referral of adult victims of domestic violence.

2. The policy must define required activities and specify who is responsible for carrying them out.

3. Hospitals must have policies and procedures that define the hospital's responsibility for collecting and safeguarding evidentiary material.

4. Medical chart documentation must include:
   - Consent from the patient, parent, or legal guardian or compliance with other applicable laws
   - Evidentiary material released by the patient

- Legally required notifications and release of information to authorities
- Referrals made to private or public community agencies for victims of abuse

13. What part does photography play in domestic violence investigation?

The importance of photography to document physical injury cannot be overemphasized. It is an important tool in both investigation and prosecution. When injuries are completely, accurately, and promptly photographed, prosecution of the batterer can occur more easily without the testimony of the victim. Victims have been coerced into not testifying by batterers. The value of a photograph is most profound when a jury or judge must review a case. With or without the victim, those photographs speak volumes about what actually happened.

14. What questions should you ask to support a forensic investigation of domestic violence?

- How many times has this happened before?
- Were you hit with closed fist or open hand?
- Were you hit with a weapon? Was a weapon present?
- Are there any marks or bruises on your body? (Do not ask about "injuries.")
- Have the children or pets been injured by the batterer before?
- You want this to stop, don't you? You want him or her to get help, don't you?
- Just tell the truth to the police and in court (Do *not* talk about testimony with the victim.)

15. What interviewing techniques can be used in domestic violence cases that present to the trauma center or emergency department?

- Separate the victim from the batterer.
- Do not allow, if possible, the two parties to hear or see one another.
- Make it easy for the victim to trust you.
- Watch your body language, tone of voice, and words.
- Look the victim in the eye.
- Do not judge the victim regardless of situation.
- Ask the right questions.
- Use calming techniques (e.g., voice tone, pace).
- Make no accusatory statements.
- Acknowledge any frustration, anger, or concern.
- Document all spontaneous remarks, and place them in quotations in the medical record.
- Interview children away from parents, if possible.
- Be at eye level with children during interview.
- Be alert to indications of fear toward any parent.
- Evaluate visually while interviewing children for signs of abuse.

16. Are photographs enough for documentation in domestic violence investigations?

No. Photographs should be augmented with a body map drawing of any and all injuries as well as a full text description of the injuries. Videotape, as permitted by protocol, is becoming a valuable tool for documentation and is used mostly by police at this time.

17. Can a digital camera be used for photographing domestic violence injury?

The answer to this question should be determined by institutional policy in conjunction with the prosecuting attorney for the jurisdiction in question. Many jurisdictions have yet to admit digital photography for court evidence. There is still some fear about preservation and authentication of digitally created works. It is highly unfortunate to have otherwise excellent photographs denied admission into court proceedings only because they are digital. This "science" is improving, however, and much progress is being made to ensure the use of digital imagery in the courts.

18. What are the key elements in the forensic investigation of a victim of domestic violence?

- Separate the victim from others, and place in a comfortable and quiet environment if possible. Limit exchange of "stories" and information between victim and suspected batterer.
- Interview and record utterances and spontaneous statements verbatim (in quotation marks).
- Ask about the possibility of weapons being held by any party present or in an area easily accessible to any party.
- Note and document victim's condition, including torn clothing, smeared makeup, and evidence of injury.
- Ask about the presence of a restraining order, and alert security or police if such an order is in effect and the restrained party is present or caused the injury (according to the victim's utterances).
- Bag the clothing of victim and batterer separately if bagging is necessary.
- Perform rape kit examination with preservation of complete chain of custody, if indicated.
- Document incident with text, photographs, and body map drawings.

19. Do I have to report an incident of domestic violence?

State law must be consulted for this answer. In many states, reporting to police of domestic violence is not mandatory by law unless the victim is disabled, elderly, or a child. In other states, certain types of injury (e.g., gun or knife wound) or injuries that result from certain events (e.g., assault, motor vehicle crash [MVC]) must be reported. In states that do not have mandatory reporting, especially when physical injury is minor or absent, reporting opens the reporter to civil risk. In domestic violence cases in a state that has no mandatory reporting requirement, without the expressed permission of the victim, reporting is not indicated even with clear evidence of domestic violence. The county or state prosecuting attorney or domestic violence police/court unit for your jurisdiction can assist in delineating which cases should be reported.

20. How may mandatory reporting be harmful?

Individual states do not mandate reporting of domestic violence for various theoretical reasons. Some have theorized that victims may refrain from seeking critically needed health care if they do not want the police called. Mandatory reporting does not respect the autonomy of victims of domestic violence. The victim of domestic violence is in most cases a competent adult who should be granted the right to make decisions that she believes will increase—not undermine—safety. Mandatory reporting also may interfere with provider-patient confidentiality and undermine patient candor and trust in the provider. Lastly, it cannot be assumed that law enforcement response will increase the safety of a battered woman. In fact, the risk may actually increase once the batterer realizes that the police "know."

21. What constitutes evidence in a domestic violence case?

- Descriptions of the condition of victim and batterer
- Condition of the crime scene (if you happen to be there), including disarray of physical surroundings (e.g., hanging art, furniture, doors)
- Photography of crime scene, victim, batterer, weapons, and surroundings
- Any possible weapons or projectiles from weapons

22. What is chain of custody? Why is it important?

Chain of custody is defined as the witnessed, written record of all persons who maintained uninterrupted control over items of evidence. It establishes proof that items of evidence collected at the crime scene (place or person) are the same items presented in the court of law. Chain of custody begins the minute that evidence is removed from the place or person involved in the crime. The initial collection, marking, and labeling begin the chain of custody and control of evidence. The chain of custody procedure documents where evidence was and where it has been. It documents who had contact with the evidence, the date and time the evidence was handled, the circumstances for handling of the evidence, and what changes, if any, were made to the evidence.

23. What information should be recorded on any evidence tag?

Information recorded on the evidence tag should be dictated primarily by the police agency of jurisdiction. In general, the evidence tag, label, or mark (depending on the item) should include a description of the item, police case or medical record number or identifier, date of collection, location of collection, collector's name and identifier, brand name of item if any, and any serial number or garment tag information. Any health care provider who is involved in evidence collection can be required to testify in court about that collection and maintenance of the chain of custody. Evidence has been "thrown out" on the basis of such testimony.

24. What is the lethality checklist? How is it applied?

A spouse or partner kills over one-half of the women killed in the U.S. every year. The lethality checklist is a list of situations and issues that, if present, indicate an increased likelihood of serious injury or death to the victim. The more items that are present, the greater the danger.

- The batterer calls the partner by a body part name.
- The batterer blames the victim for injuries.
- The batterer is unwilling to turn the victim lose.
- The batterer shows an obsession with the victim.
- The batterer is hostile and angry.
- The batterer or victim mentions suicide or has a history of a suicide attempt.
- The batterer shows extreme jealousy.
- The victim is blamed for a variety of promiscuous behaviors.
- Previous violent incidents have occurred.
- The batterer has killed or injured pets at home.
- Threats have been or are being made by either party.
- The batterer has access to victim.
- The batterer has access to guns.
- Alcohol, amphetamines, cocaine, or methamphetamine is involved.
- The batterer indicates the desire to hurt the partner.
- The batterer expresses no desire to stop the violence or control behavior.

25. What is the future of domestic violence treatment?

Stopping domestic violence requires a coordinated community response in which health care providers, criminal justice systems, domestic violence shelters, and social service agencies join forces. This multifaceted problem requires a community effort. Clearly, nursing triage and assessment in the outpatient facility are key factors.

ELDER ABUSE

26. What is included in the crime of elder abuse?

Physical violence, psychological and emotional abuse (threats, verbal abuse, violation of basic privacy), financial or legal exploitation, and neglect (failure to meet basic needs) are included, either together or apart, in elder abuse.

27. What are the most common characteristics of a victim of elder abuse?

The victim of elder abuse is likely to be older than 70 years, female, dependent on the abuser in some manner for support (e.g., finances, basic needs, ambulation, transportation), and suffering from a debilitating mental or physical illness.

28. What are the most common features of elder abusers?

The abuser of the elderly is likely to be stressed or strained from caring for an older person. This stress can cause frustration and increases the likelihood of abuse. Substance abuse (alcohol or drugs) may play a role in increasing the likelihood of elder abuse. If the abuser is dependent on the victim for food, clothing, or shelter, the possibility of violence increases when stress/strain or substance abuse is present.

29. What are the possible signs of neglect in the elderly?

Signs of abuse and neglect in the elderly can include failure to receive adequate medical and dental care, drug or alcohol abuse in the victim, poor general hygiene and basic care (skin lesions are common), chronic fatigue or listlessness with previous history of active lifestyle, and malnutrition or dehydration.

30. Why does elder abuse continue once it starts?

There are many reasons for continued elderly abuse. The older person who feels dependent on the abuser may fear loss of care if the abuser is arrested or removed. If the older person has physical or mental illness, reporting is less likely.

31. What resources in the community may be of assistance in caring for the elderly and preventing elder abuse when frustration and strain are present?

Community resources include daily home visits by professional caregivers, support organizations and groups, counseling services, transportation services, meal preparation and delivery services, day care, and long-term residential facilities. In many cases of elder abuse, families were unaware of such services.

CHILD ABUSE

32. What are some of the physical signs or indicators of child abuse?

Physical indications of child abuse can include bite marks (an adult bite mark must be greater than 3–4 cm canine [canine measurement]), drug abuse in parent with or without history of drug use during pregnancy, spiral long bone fractures in children under the age of 2–3 years, unexplained injuries or burns (cigarette burns), and injuries inconsistent with the reported history.

33. What are some of the more common signs of sexual abuse in children?

Any one or combination of the following physical manifestations should alert the clinician to the possibility of sexual abuse: bruising or bleeding of the genitalia, perineum, or perianal area; recurrent urinary tract infection; sexually transmitted disease; vaginal discharge; torn or bloody clothing; or difficult or painful sitting or walking.

34. What are the requirements for reporting child abuse?

In most states, all known or suspected cases of child abuse, neglect, or abandonment must be reported to the state or local agency involved in child and family services. In many states, a hotline number is available for initial contact with the agency or on-call case manager. In cases of severe injury, sexual abuse, or other criminal offense, it also may be necessary to contact local law enforcement. It is imperative to understand state, local, and institutional policy and procedure before the event occurs. Contact your local state attorney and/or child crimes investigator.

35. What type of forensic evidence should be collected for child abuse cases?

Largely what is collected and how it is collected should be guided by established procedures determined by the institution in cooperation with local law enforcement, prosecutors, and judges. Collection focuses on three main types of forensic evidence:

1. Identification evidence of victim, batterer, and injuries (including photographs, body maps, text descriptions)

2. Behavioral evidence of victim and batterer (if present), including videotape and text description

3. Biologic evidence (e.g., specimen), when present

In general, the best medical forensic evidence is based on clear documentation of the history and physical examination, accurate body map description of injury and wounds, and clear photographs (close-ups, medium shots, and long shots at a far distance from injuries and victim). If videotape is permitted or court-ordered, it can be extremely helpful to document not only identification and injury but also victim behavior.

36. What are the essential basics of documentation?

- Site and time of assault
- Identification of assailant or batterer
- Relationship of victim to assailant or batterer
- Weapons and restraints used
- What actually took place (mechanism of injury or assault)
- Activities of the victim that may have destroyed evidence
- Victim's general appearance and response during exam
- Physical injuries

37. Describe the process of forensic evidence processing.

Forensic procedures demand attention to proper collection (including description, packaging, labeling, photographs, and diagrams of sites), proper transportation and storage (including chain of evidence), proper processing and testing in the crime or medical lab, and proper reporting, including interpretation and report accuracy.

38. Define forensics.

Forensics relates to the use of science or technology in the investigation and establishment of facts or evidence in a court of law. Forensic medicine deals with the identification, collection, and processing of facts and evidence from occurrences related to human physiology and anatomy in health and disease or injury.

39. What type of evidence is considered to be forensic evidence?

The field of forensic evidence is growing daily. Currently evidence categories considered forensic include the following:

- Botany (plant material)
- Pathology (DNA and biologic tissue)
- Documents and handwriting
- Drugs and toxicology
- Entomology (insect materials)
- Standard prints (finger, hand, other body parts)
- Firearms, weapons, and ballistics
- Impressions (footprint, tire tracks)
- Trace evidence (hair, fibers, dried blood, gun powder)
- Anthropology (origin and physical, social, and cultural development of humans)
- Computer materials (digital data, software, hardware)
- Behavioral profiling (forensic psychiatry or psychology)

40. What is the position of the Emergency Nurses Association in regard to forensic evidence collection?

• Believes that it is the nurse's role not only to provide physical and emotional care to patients but also to help preserve the chain of evidence collected in the emergency department.

• Supports collaboration with emergency physicians, social service, and law enforcement personnel to develop guidelines for forensic evidence collection and documentation in the emergency care setting.

• Encourages nurses to become familiar with the concepts and skills of evidence collection and photographic and written documentation.

BIBLIOGRAPHY

1. Augenbraun M, Wilson TE, Allister L: Domestic violence reported by women attending a sexually transmitted disease clinic. Sex Transm Dis 28:143–147, 2001.
2. Barthauer L: Domestic violence in the psychiatric emergency service. New Dir Ment Health Serv 82:29–42, 1999.
3. Brenneman K: Forensic nursing teaches nurses to preserve evidence. Boston Bus J 17(40):12, 1997.
4. Clapp L: Ending domestic violence is everyone's responsibility: An integrated approach to domestic violence treatment. Nurs Clin North Am 35(2):481–488, 2000.
5. Davies K, Edwards L: Domestic violence: A challenge to accident and emergency nurses. Accid Emerg Nurs 7:26–30, 1999.
6. Freed PE, Drake VK: Mandatory reporting of abuse: Practical, moral, and legal issues for psychiatric home healthcare nurses. Issues Ment Health Nurs 20:423–436, 1999.
7. Emergency Nurses Association Position Statement: Forensic evidence collection. J Emerg Nurs 24(5):38A, 1998.
8. Garbacz-Bader DM: Forensic science program: A community effort. Am J Forens Med Pathol 19(3):242–245, 1997.
9. Grunfeld AF, Ritmiller S, Mackay K, et al: Detecting domestic violence against women in the emergency department: A nursing triage model. J Emerg Nurs 20(4):271–274, 1994.
10. Guth AA, Pachter L: Domestic violence and the trauma surgeon. Am J Surg 179(2):134–140, 2000.
11. Haywood YC, Haile-Mariam T: Violence against women. Emerg Med Clin North Am 17(3):603–615, 1999.
12. Jensen LA: The cycle of domestic violence and the barriers to treatment. Nurse Pract 25(5):26, 29, 2000.
13. Jezierski MB, Eickholt T, McGee J: Disadvantages to mandatory reporting of domestic violence. J Emerg Nurs 25(2):79–80, 1999.
14. McConnell EA: Myths and facts about domestic violence. Nursing 30(4):69, 2000.
15. Morewitz SJ: Domestic violence and stalking during pregnancy. Obstet Gynecol 97(suppl 1):S53, 2001.
16. Patterson MM: Child abuse: Assessment and intervention. Orthop Nurs 17:49–54; quiz , 55–56, 1998.
17. Roberts GL, O'Toole BI, Lawrence JM, Raphael B: Domestic violence victims in a hospital emergency department. Med J Aust 159(5):307–310, 1993.
18. Ross MM, Hoff LA, Coutu-Wakulczyk G: Nursing curricula and violence issues. J Nurs Educ 37(2):53–60, 1998.
19. Saunder EE: Screening for domestic violence during pregnancy. Int J Trauma Nurs 6(2):44–47, 2000.
20. Scheller TF, Berens P: Domestic violence and substance use. Obstet Gynecol 97(4 Suppl 1):S53, 2001.
21. Sirotnak SP, Sorotnak AP: Child abuse and forensic pediatric medicine fellowship curriculum statement. Child Maltreat 5(1):58–63, 2000.
22. Tilden VP, Shepherd P: Increasing the rate of identification of battered women in an emergency department: Use of a nursing protocol. Res Nurs Health 10(4):209–215, 1987.
23. Tillett J, Hanson L: Midwifery triage and management of trauma and second/third trimester bleeding. J Nurse Midwifery 44(5):439–448, 1999.
24. Williams-Evans SA, Evans KR, Call-Schmidt T, Williams G: The lived experiences of adult female victims of child abuse. J Cult Divers 7(2):48–54, 2000.

Websites

25. DMOZ Open Directory Project on Domestic Violence: http://dmoz.org/Society/People/Women/ Issues/Domestic_Violence/.
26. Women in Distress of Broward County Florida: http://www.womenindistress.org/.
27. Florida Domestic Violence Task Force: http://www5.myflorida.com/cf_web/myflorida/healthfamily/ learn/familyissues/domesticviolence/.
28. Domestic Violence Shelters in the U.S. (listing): http://www.sboard.org/SHELTERS.HTM
29. Emergency Nurses Association: http://www.ena.org/.
30. Rural Health Response to Domestic Violence: Policy and Practice Issues Health Resources Services Administration (HRSA); U.S. Dept. of Health and Human Resources: http://www.ruralhealth. hrsa.gov/domviol.htm.
31. United State Department of Justice: Domestic Violence: http://www.usdoj.gov/domesticviolence.htm.
32. U.S. Office of Personnel Management on Domestic Violence: http://www.opm.gov/ehs\workplac\ html\domestic.html.
33. National Domestic Violence Hotline: http://www.ndvh.org/ (1-800-799-SAFE [7233]).
34. Family Violence Prevention Fund - Routine Screening Recommendations 1999: http://www.fvpf. org/health/screpol.pdf.

18. TOXICOLOGY

Joe Spillane, PharmD, ABAT

1. Which drug of abuse is most commonly involved in trauma cases?

Alcohol is clearly the most commonly involved drug of abuse in trauma cases. Alcohol is estimated to be associated with 40–50% of traffic fatalities, 25–35% of all nonfatal traffic accidents, up to 64% of all fires and burns, 40% of all falls, approximately 50% of all homicides (victim or perpetrator), and 47% of nontraffic accident fatalities.

2. How do alcohol abusers increase their risk for trauma?

1. The alcohol abuser is more likely to experience trauma than a sober person.

2. Clinical manifestations of trauma, especially head injuries, can be masked or mimicked by intoxication with alcohol, leading to over- or underdiagnosing.

3. Alcohol can further complicate the management of trauma because of concerns of the interactions between alcohol and medications. For example, surgery may be delayed because of concerns with anesthesia in a patient with high alcohol levels. Indeed, alcoholics tend to regurgitate and aspirate stomach contents during anesthesia.

3. Are intoxicated persons less likely to be hurt or killed in an accident because they are so relaxed?

Although there are some exceptions, most research shows that, given similar traumatic circumstances, a drinker is likely to sustain a more serious injury than a nondrinker. The exact mechanism is not clear, but the belief that intoxicated persons are less likely to be hurt or killed is probably a myth.

4. Discuss the usefulness of obtaining an alcohol level in the trauma patient with altered mental status.

An alcohol level is useful in the trauma patient for the following reasons:

1. It can give a rough idea of how much of the altered mental status may be due to alcohol as opposed to some coexisting condition.

2. A reasonably coherent person with a high alcohol level or a person in withdrawal should be referred for appropriate alcohol treatment.

5. How should an alcohol level be interpreted in trauma patients?

Blood alcohol (ethanol) levels of 20–60 mg/dl (0.02–0.06%) in most nontolerant people reduce inhibitions (causing the person to take more risks) and anxiety and impair ability to perform complex or recently learned tasks. In most states, legal intoxication is defined as 80 mg/dl (0.08%). Depending on individual tolerance, higher levels can progress from slowed reaction time to ataxia to slurred speech, confusion, unresponsiveness, coma, and respiratory failure. Most alcohol-induced fatalities occur at levels above 400 mg/dl.

6. How quickly is alcohol metabolized?

Alcohol is generally metabolized at the rate of 15–25 mg/dl/hour; in a heavy drinker, the rate may increase to 40 mg/dl/hour.

7. Is a toxicology screen a good way to rule out a toxicologic cause of altered mental status in a trauma patient?

No. There are thousands of potential intoxicants, and most urine toxicology screens performed in hospitals test only for 5 or 6 categories of drugs (usually drugs of abuse). Knowing this limitation, it should be obvious that even the most comprehensive of available hospital toxicology screens cannot rule out the possibility of a toxicologic cause. In addition, the fact that a person tests positive for a certain drug or chemical in the urine (provided no errors have been made) certainly does not mean that that drug or chemical is causing the clinical manifestations. In addition, the health care team may have given the agent as a treatment; therefore, it is not part of the problem. For example, a toxicologic screen for benzodiazepine may be positive after the patient is intubated with the rapid-sequence intubation (RSI) method. A benzodiazepine is commonly used with RSI. In addition, many toxicologic screens detect only the metabolite, not the parent compound. Indeed, for the average laboratory, the rate of false-negative results is 10–30%, whereas the rate of false-positive results is 0–10%.

8. Do most hospital toxicology screens at least detect the most common intoxicants?
No. Examples of common intoxicants that are not commonly detected on most "comprehensive screens" include gamma hydroxybutyrate (GHB), lysergic acid diethylamide (LSD), clonidine, digoxin, lithium, fentanyl, ketamine (Special K), flunitrazepam (roofies), methadone, designer opiates, iron, organophosphates, and many newer and other drugs and chemicals. Even if the screens detect an intoxicant that was not expected, it is exceedingly rare that that information would or should significantly change management.

9. How can one tell whether drug toxicity is responsible for altered mental status in a trauma patient?
The diagnosis lies in the physical exam and complete history. A properly interpreted blood alcohol level and urine toxicology screen may provide some help but almost certainly will not provide the whole answer.

10. Which clues on physical exam may help to distinguish toxicologic vs. traumatic causes of altered mental status?
Focal findings (asymmetry of cranial nerves, motor strength, reflexes, and eye findings) are extremely unlikely if altered mental status is due to a purely toxicologic cause; a structural lesion is much more likely to be responsible. Most overdoses result in symmetrical findings. Obviously needle marks and/or the presence of drug paraphernalia are important clues. In addition, the presence of toxidromes or constellations of signs, symptoms, and lab values that are characteristic of certain overdoses are important to note.

11. What are some common toxidromes?
The classic triad of hypotension, central nervous system depression (respiratory depression), and pinpoint pupils is consistent with **opioid or clonidine** intoxication. **Salicylates** can cause tachypnea or hyperpnea with a high anion gap metabolic acidosis. **Cocaine** or any sympathomimetic can cause tachycardia, hyperthermia, hypertension, tremor, diaphoresis, agitation, and large pupils. **Anticholinergics** cause tachycardia, hyperthermia, agitation, and mydriasis similar to sympathomimetics but are usually accompanied by flushed dry skin and, potentially, hallucinations.

12. Describe a reasonable management approach to the trauma patient with altered mental status who may have coexisting drug toxicity.
As with any patient, symptomatic/supportive care is paramount, including rapid evaluation of blood glucose. A dose of naloxone (pure opioid antagonist) may be diagnostic and therapeutic. An alcohol level should be obtained and interpreted. A comprehensive history (when obtainable) should include any information about the possibility of a drug overdose or withdrawal. This information can be forwarded to the lab if a urine toxicology screen is warranted. Thiamine is also reasonable to prevent and treat Wernicke's encephalopathy. Further consultation with a poison center and/or clinical toxicologist is also helpful.

BIBLIOGRAPHY

1. Feske S: Neurologic emergencies, coma and confusional states: Emergency department diagnosis and management. Neurol Clin 16:238–257, 1998.
2. Gallagher EJ, Lewin NA: Neurologic principles. In Goldfrank L, et al (eds): Goldfrank's Toxicologic Emergencies, 6th ed. Stamford, CT, Appleton & Lange, 1998, pp 309–336.
3. Hoffman RS, Goldfrank LR: The poisoned patient with altered consciousness: Controversies in the use of a "coma cocktail." JAMA 274:562–569, 1995.
4. Huth J, et al: Effects of accurate ethanolism on the hospital course and outcome of injured automobile drivers. J Trauma 23:494–498, 1983.
5. Lowenfels A, Miller T: Alcohol and trauma. Ann Emerg Med 13:1056–1060, 1984.
6. National Institute on Alcohol Abuse and Alcoholism (NIAAA): Alcohol and trauma. Alcohol Alert No. 3, January 1989.
7. Osterloh JD: Laboratory testing in emergency toxicology. In Ford M, et al (eds): Clinical Toxicology. Philadelphia, Saunders, 2001, pp 51–60.
8. Ward R, et al: Effects of ethanol on the severity and outcome of trauma. Am J Surg 144:153–157, 1982.

19. ORGAN DONATION AND ORGAN PROCUREMENT

Mary-Ellen Anton, RN, BSN, MHM, CCRN, CPTC

1. Discuss the current crisis in organ transplantation.

The current crisis in transplantation is due simply to a matter of supply and demand. In 2002, for example, 78,000 people were on the national waiting list. Unfortunately, over the past decade or so, only 5,000–6,000 patients donate organs each year. As technology improves and medical advances increase, more and more people survive to end-stage organ failure and are entered onto the waiting lists. The organs necessary to save their lives are not available, and many people die while waiting for their organ transplant.

2. What is the major challenge in organ donation and transplantation?

To procure successfully the organs so desperately needed to save the lives of patients awaiting transplant.

3. What are the different categories of donation?

1. **Brain-dead donor.** Brain death has been pronounced. The patient is maintained hemodynamically and has total ventilatory support.

2. **Living related donor.** Living person chooses to donate a kidney or portion of his or her liver or lung to another person. Often the recipient is a family member (e.g., a father donates a kidney to his son).

3. **Non–heart-beating donor.** The patient has minimal neurologic function but is not brain dead, and family members have decided to withdraw life support. With a procurement team present, organ rescue begins after pronouncement of death by cardiac arrest (asystole must occur within 15–30 minutes of extubation for organs to remain viable for transplant).

4. **Post-cardiopulmonary arrest patient.** The patient's death is pronounced by cessation of cardiopulmonary function. (Because of prolonged absence of both perfusion and ventilation, organs are not viable for transplantation.)

4. What are the criteria for donation of organs or tissues?

The criteria for donation may differ from organ procurement organization (OPO) to OPO or region to region. In general, patients with human immunodeficiency virus (HIV), active hepatitis B, or communicable diseases such as active tuberculosis are excluded. Age limits or restrictions also vary. The criteria, however, for who can donate are always being expanded. Never rule out a patient as a potential donor until the local OPO is consulted.

5. Does a diagnosis of active hepatitis exclude a patient from donation?

Generally active hepatitis B rules out donation. Patients with other types of hepatitis (A, C, D, or E) or hepatitis B antibodies are not necessarily ruled out. Confer with your local OPO.

6. Which organs and tissues can be donated?

Brain-dead organ donor: organs, eyes, bone, tissue*
Living related donor: kidney, lobe of liver, portion of lung*
Non–heart-beating donor: abdominal organs, eyes, tissue*
Cardiac arrest donor: eyes, bone, tissue*

* Dependent on local OPO determination of criteria for donation.

7. What are the current laws and regulations governing organ donation in the United States?

1. Omnibus Reconciliation Act of 1986 (Required Request/Routine Inquiry): law requires hospitals to have processes in place that ensure that all families of potential donors are offered the option of organ and/or tissue donation at or near the time of death.

2. Health Care Finance Administration (HCFA) 3005-F: effective in 1998, this regulation requires the following:
- Hospitals must participate with local OPO, eye, and bone bank.
- Hospitals must report all deaths to local OPO.
- Triage of potential donors must be done by OPO, not by hospital staff.
- Only trained requestors may approach families with the donation option.

8. Can a trauma patient or other patients requiring a medical examiner's or coroner's autopsy still donate?

Guidelines may vary from state to state, but the medical examiner's approval is required for any donation that falls within his or her jurisdiction. Autopsy, however, does not preclude donation.

9. What is brain death?

In the United States, brain death is legally defined as the total cessation of brain and brainstem function.

10. What brainstem reflexes are usually tested when an assessment for brain death is performed?

The common tests for brainstem function include, but are not limited to, the following:
- Pain response
- Pupillary response
- Apnea
- Vestibulo-ocular reflex response (caloric ice water test)
- Oculocephalic reflex response (doll's eyes)
- Facial sensory and motor response (absence of corneal and jaw reflexes)
- Pharyngeal and tracheal reflex response (absence of cough and gag reflexes)

11. Two physicians have documented on the chart that the patient meets the clinical criteria for brain death. During routine care, the patient suddenly takes a single breath independently of the ventilator. Is the patient brain-dead?

No. Spontaneous respirations indicate some function of the respiratory center in the brainstem.

12. Is an electroencephalogram, nuclear brain flow study, or cerebral angiography necessary for the pronouncement of death?

Requirements may vary from state to state and hospital to hospital. In most states, confirmatory testing is not mandatory and brain death can be pronounced by clinical evaluation only.

13. How many physicians must document absence of cardiopulmonary function for legal pronouncement of cardiac death?

One.

14. How many physicians must document clinical brain death for legal pronouncement of death?

Two.

15. When is the best time to approach the patient's family with the option of organ donation?
Generally, after they have been informed and are accepting of the death.

16. Who should approach the family?
According to the 1998 HCFA requirements, the person approaching a family with the option of organ donation must be trained to do so. Local OPOs provide this training. Studies have shown that donation increases by almost 50% when an OPO coordinator is involved.

17. How should the family be approached?
With compassion and caring. Families must be given the information that they need to make an informed decision about donation.

18. Define decoupling.
Decoupling is the separation of the announcement of death and the approach to the family about organ donation. Research has shown that families require a period of adjustment to the fact that death has occurred. If they are approached too quickly or at the same time that they are told of the death, only 47% of families will say "yes" to donation. If decoupling is used, consent rises to 78%.

19. What is the preferred setting in which to approach the family?
A private, quiet, nonthreatening environment, away from the patient's bedside. Simply providing privacy can increase donation by 24%.

20. Can a family say "no" to donation even if the deceased has a valid donor card or driver's license designation?
Many state statutes state that no one can refute a properly executed donor card. Most OPOs, however, defer to the family's decision or wishes.

21. List three issues that potential donor families commonly fear and need to know before they can make an informed decision about organ and tissue donation.
1. There is no cost to donation.
2. Their loved one will not experience pain or suffering.
3. There is no disfigurement with donation.

22. What two steps must take place before procurement activities can begin?
Consent for donation and documentation of death.

23. What elements are involved in the procurement/donation process?
1. Documentation of death
2. Consent from next-of-kin and continued emotional support of family
3. Donor evaluation and hemodynamic maintenance
4. Organ evaluation
5. Placement of organs (locating suitable recipients)
6. Surgical rescue of organs and tissues
7. Preservation of organs and tissues
8. Transportation of organs/tissues to waiting recipients
9. Aftercare of donor families

24. What is the "rule of 100"?
A set of simplified goals for the maintenance of a potential organ donor:
• Systolic blood pressure > 100 mmHg (maintenance of adequate organ perfusion)
• Urine output > 100 ml/hr (maintenance of renal perfusion)
• Pulse oxygenation > 100% (maintenance of adequate ventilation and oxygenation)

25. What tests are done to evaluate the various organs for suitability for transplantation?

ORGAN	TEST/EXAM
Heart	Cardiac enzymes, electrocardiogram (ECG) Echocardiogram (if ECG within normal limits) Cardiac catheterization (if patient is older than 40 years and echocardiogram is within normal limits)
Lungs	Arterial blood gases, oxygen challenge, chest x-rays Bronchoscopy (if arterial blood gases and chest x-ray are within normal limits) with acid-fast bacillus test and culture and sensitivities
Liver	Biochemical profile, liver panel, and function studies (possible bedside liver biopsy if history or age dictates)
Kidneys	Blood urea nitrogen, creatinine, urinalysis
Pancreas	Amylase, lipase, and blood sugar

26. Is there more than one list for recipients?

There is one national list, but it can be subdivided into regional and local lists. Recipients are usually entered locally by the transplant centers where they are listed and hope to be transplanted.

27. How do we know that the most critical/deserving patient gets the organ and that someone rich or famous does not get priority?

The national list is maintained by the United Network for Organ Sharing (UNOS), a non-profit organization in Virginia that is responsible for overseeing the equitable distribution of organs in the U.S. The list is computer-generated based on numerical classifications for all potential recipients.

28. What criteria are used to determine a patient's priority on the national list?

The criteria include, but are not limited to, the following:
• Severity of illness
• Blood type
• Height and weight
• Geographic location
• HLA matching for pancreas and kidneys
• Length of time waiting

29. How long is the entire donation process?

The entire donation process, from consent to conclusion of surgery, can take from 8 to more than 24 hours.

30. Does the donation process interfere with the family's funeral arrangements?

Most OPOs work continuously throughout the day and night, and generally the procurement is completed without adding extra time to the family's plans for viewings or funerals.

31. What happens to the patient during the long period of evaluation and maintenance?

The patient is hemodynamically maintained, and all necessary testing (see question 25) is completed. With occasional exceptions, most testing can be completed at the bedside. The ventilator, intravenous lines, and all care and treatments needed to sustain the patient are continued.

32. When is the ventilator discontinued?

In the operating room.

33. A patient is pronounced brain-dead at 11 AM. If the ventilator is turned off in the operating room and asystole occurs at 6 AM the following morning, what is the official time of death?

11 AM. Brain death is medical and legal death.

34. What guarantees are made to the donor family?

The only guarantees that are made to the family is that their loved one will be treated with the utmost respect and dignity throughout the procurement process.

35. How is the patient prepared for surgery?

A complete shave of the patient's chest and abdomen from neck to groin is necessary. A scrub preparation (usually with povidone-iodine) is completed for the same area before the patient is draped for surgery.

36. How long can organs remain out of body before they must be transplanted?

ORGAN	PERIOD OF VIABILITY OUTSIDE THE BODY
Heart/lung	4–6 hours
Liver	12 hours
Pancreas	12 hours
Intestines	12 hours
Kidneys	24–72 hours

37. During surgery, what determines the final acceptance of the organ for donation?

Visualization of the organ by the procuring surgeon.

38. What factors must the procurement coordinator take into consideration when scheduling a time for the surgery?

- Family needs, restrictions, limitations
- Stability of donor
- Availability of operating room
- Availability of procurement surgeons and staff
- Ability of transplant center to locate and have recipient ready to receive the organ for transplant as soon as possible after recovery of organs

39. What happens to the body postoperatively?

After the procurement, the incision is surgically closed as in any other type of surgery. The body is prepared for the medical examiner and/or funeral home, wrapped in an appropriate shroud, and typically taken to the morgue.

40. Who pays the expenses incurred during the donation?

All expenses incurred during the donation process are the responsibility of the OPO. The donor family or donor's estate does not pay for any of the expenses of the donation. The OPO cannot, however, pay for any treatments or costs incurred while trying to save the patient's life or prior to the death pronouncement.

41. Can the OPO pay for funeral expenses?

Although this rule may be changing soon, currently the OPO is not permitted to pay for funeral expenses in most states. Consult local statutes.

42. Do the donor families get to meet the recipients?

It has been against the policy of many OPOs to facilitate the meeting. These restrictions are being challenged throughout the country, and progressive changes may be forthcoming. Many OPOs, however, furnish donor families with nonidentifying information about the recipients, such as age, sex, and city of residency.

43. What is donor family aftercare?

Although the name of the service may vary, most OPOs provide some type of donor family care after donation. This care may include, but is not limited to, availability of support groups, donor family support activities, bereavement literature, and social service referrals.

44. What are the benefits of donation to recipients?

They receive the gift of life.

45. What are the benefits of donation to the trauma nurse?

A chance to be a part of the continuation of care to the donor patients and their families and the opportunity to help provide these families with something positive in their darkest hours.

46. What are the benefits to the donor family?

The knowledge that their loved one "lives on" in others through organ and tissue donation greatly assists many families in dealing with grief and loss. Many take comfort and solace in knowing that others were saved and now live because of the donor's precious gifts.

CONTROVERSIES AND MYTHS

47. Describe the urban legend of the bathtub kidney donation. Is it true?

After a young man is seduced in a cocktail lounge and unknowingly drugged, his kidney is removed. The young man awakens to find himself in a bathtub full of ice with a sign that reads, "Call 911. Your kidney has been removed."

In reality, all donations in the United States occur in controlled hospital-based settings. Medical and social histories and family consent, as well as serology testing, are obtained before the organ is procured in a sterile operating room. UNOS is involved to ensure equitable allocation of every rescued organ in the United States. Unfortunately, stories of "black marketing" of organs outside the borders of the United States are heard frequently. Fact or fiction, organs procured in this fashion are not used within the United States.

48. Describe the urban legend of baby snatching for organs. Is it true?

A child is kidnapped and subsequently murdered for organs.

In reality, this scenario does not happen in United States. As stated above, all donations occur in hospitals with OPO and UNOS involvement. Full disclosure of past and present social and medical histories is necessary. Donors are brain-dead, with consent from families, known histories, serologies, and other test results.

49. Is there any truth to the urban legend that rescue workers, doctors, and nurses will not try to save your life if they know that you have a donor card?

Absolutely not. In a life-threatening medical emergency, everything is done to save the patient's life. Donation and the existence of a donor card are never a consideration until brain death or cardiac death has occurred.

50. What about the belief that asking about donation will only cause the family more pain?

Health care professionals commonly cite this fear as a reason for reluctance to approach families about donation at or near the time of the patient's death. Families who have donated report that being approached with the option is neither an intrusion on their grief nor an invasion of their privacy. In fact, most state that they are grateful that someone cared enough to offer the option.

51. True or false: If health care professionals know that you have a donor card, they will take your organs before you are dead.

False. No one is murdered in the United States to procure organs for donation.

52. True or false: I can sell my own organs anytime I want.

False. It is illegal in the United States to buy or sell organs on computer auctions or by any other method.

53. True or false: If you are famous, you can get to the top of the waiting list.

Rumors that wealthy or famous people such as Mickey Mantle and Larry Hagman get priority on the waiting list are common. In reality, the national transplant waiting list is computerized. People are given priority based on matching blood type, tissue typing, size, height, weight, and geographical location. Children are also given priority. UNOS is a nonprofit organization that oversees and ensures the equitable allocation of organs in the U.S. Wealth or fame does not ensure that a transplantable organ will be available.

BIBLIOGRAPHY

1. Ehrle RN, et al: Referral, request and consent for organ donation: Best practice—A blueprint for success. Crit Care Nurse 9(2):21–33, 1999.
2. Medicare and Medicaid Programs: Hospital conditions of participation; provider agreements and supplier approval, 42 CFR Part 482. 62 Federal Register, 1997.
3. Sullivan J, et al: Determining brain death. Crit Care Nurs 19(2):37–46, 1999.
4. United Network for Organ Sharing (UNOS), Richmond VA: Waiting list/transplant data and statistics. Available at www.UNOS.org. Accessed January, 2002.
5. University of Miami Organ Procurement Organization: Educational materials and protocol book, 1998.

INDEX

Entries in **boldface type** indicate complete chapters.

American Red Cross, 57
American Society for Testing and Materials, 38
Aminophylline, as anaphylactic shock treatment, 113
Ammonia burns, ocular, 70
Amniotic fluid embolus, 127
Amputated body parts, replantation of, 100, 105
Amputations, traumatic, 100, 104
  of the ear, 70
  electrical trauma-related, 123
  incomplete differentiated from complete, 105
Amylase, as pancreatic injury indicator, 89
Analgesics, use in pregnant trauma patients, 128
Anaphylactic shock, 112–113
Anemia, secondary brain injury-related, 64
Anesthesia, for emergency wound suturing, 99
Aneurysm, abdominal aortic, rupture of, 91
Angiography, cerebral, for brain death confirmation, 156
Animal bites, 9
Anterior chamber, blood in, 70
Anterior cord syndrome, 72
Anterior fossa fractures, 61
Anthrax, 18, 19
Antibiotic prophylaxis, in burn patients, 119
Anticholinergics, adverse effects of, 152
Anticonvulsants, as traumatic brain injury treatment, 66
Antihistamines, as anaphylactic shock treatment, 113
Anxiolytic agents, use in pain management, 120
Aorta
  retroperitoneal location of, 93
  rib fracture-related injury to, 81
  tears or dissections of, 78, 82
Asphalt burns, 120
Asphyxiation, 18
Aspirin, effect on coagulation, 103
Assaults, 26
Asystole, electrical trauma-related, 123
Atelectasis
  cervical spine injury-related, 74
  drowning-related, 133
  methylprednisolone-related, 73
  in pediatric trauma patients, 133
  splenectomy-related, 88
  traumatic brain injury-related, 67
Atrial fibrillation, electrical trauma-related, 123
Atropine
  as nerve agent exposure treatment, 21
  use in pediatric rapid-sequence induction intubation, 131
Auscultation, abdominal, 85
Autonomic dysfunction, 63
Autonomy, of patients, 114
Autopsy, implication for organ donation, 156
Avulsion injuries, 96, 104
  hepatic, 87
Axial loading, 9

"Baby snatching," for organ donations, 160
BAC (blood alcohol concentration), 32, 151

Bacillus anthracis, 18
Bag-valve devices, 83
Barbiturates, as severe traumatic brain injury treatment, 65
Bathrooms
  fall prevention in, 53
  as scald burn site, 54
Battering. *See* Domestic violence and abuse
Battle sign, 61
Beck's triad, in cardiac tamponade, 81
Benzodiazepines, toxicology screen for, 152
Beta blockers, effect on hypovolemic shock-related tachycardia, 110, 137
Betadine (povidone-iodine solution), as wound cleansing agent, 105–106
Bicycle accidents, in children, 37, 39, 129
  duodenal hematomas associated with, 90
Bicycle helmets, 37–38
Bicycle Helmet Safety Institute, 38
Bicycle safety, 37–40
Biomechanics and mechanism, of injury, **7–11**
Bioterrorism, **17–24**
Bite marks, child abuse-related, 146
Bite wounds, 104
Bladder, rupture of, 8, 93
Blast pressure, 21
Blood
  banked, 2,3-diphosphoglyceric acid deficiency of, 110
  from hemothorax, autotransfusion of, 79
  in nasogastric aspirate, 90
  at the urethral meatus, 93
Blood alcohol concentration (BAC), 32, 151
Blood flow
  assessment of, in the extremities, 96
  uterine, 125
Blood loss. *See also* Hemorrhage
  in children, 129
Blood pressure. *See also* Hypertension; Hypotension
  pain-related increase in, 120
  systolic, in compartment syndrome, 95
Blood transfusions
  autotransfusions, with blood from hemothorax, 79
  as hypovolemic shock treatment, 110
  Jehovah's Witnesses' refusal of, 114
Blunt trauma, 7
  abdominal, 85
    in children, 131
    as compartment syndrome cause, 91
    diverting colostomy in, 107
  cardiac, fatal, 82
  cervical, 71
  in children, 129, 131
    as cardiopulmonary arrest cause, 134
  in combination with penetrating trauma, 10
  electrical trauma-related, 123
  gastric, 88
  injury mechanisms of, 7
  pancreatic, 89
  splenic, 87–88
  thoracic, 77, 78